SET THE EARTH ON FIRE

SET THE EARTH ON FIRE

THE GREAT ANTHRACITE COAL STRIKE OF 1902 AND THE BIRTH OF THE POLICE

DAVID CORREIA

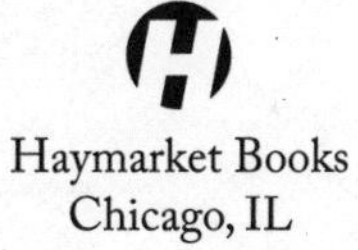

Haymarket Books
Chicago, IL

Published in 2024 by
Haymarket Books
P.O. Box 180165
Chicago, IL 60618
www.haymarketbooks.org

ISBN: 979-8-88890-090-1

Distributed to the trade in the US through Consortium Book Sales and Distribution (www.cbsd.com) and internationally through Ingram Publisher Services International (www.ingramcontent.com).

This book was published with the generous support of Lannan Foundation, Wallace Action Fund, and Marguerite Casey Foundation.

Cover and interior design by Eric Kerl.

Printed in Canada by union labor.

Library of Congress Cataloging-in-Publication data is available.

10 9 8 7 6 5 4 3 2

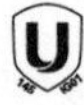

May God above
Send down a dove
With wings as sharp as razors
To cut the throats
Of those old bloats
Who take the miners' wages

CONTENTS

Preface IX

Introduction: Dig Another Grave 1

1. A Good Practical Miner 15
2. A Miners' Timeline 43
3. On Strike Day in Hazleton 73
4. They Called It the Flying Squadron 101
5. The Occupation of Shenandoah 129
6. The Jeddo Evictions 149
7. Show Us the Lung of a Miner 161

Conclusion: A Wrecking Crew 181

Acknowledgments 195

References 197

Index 267

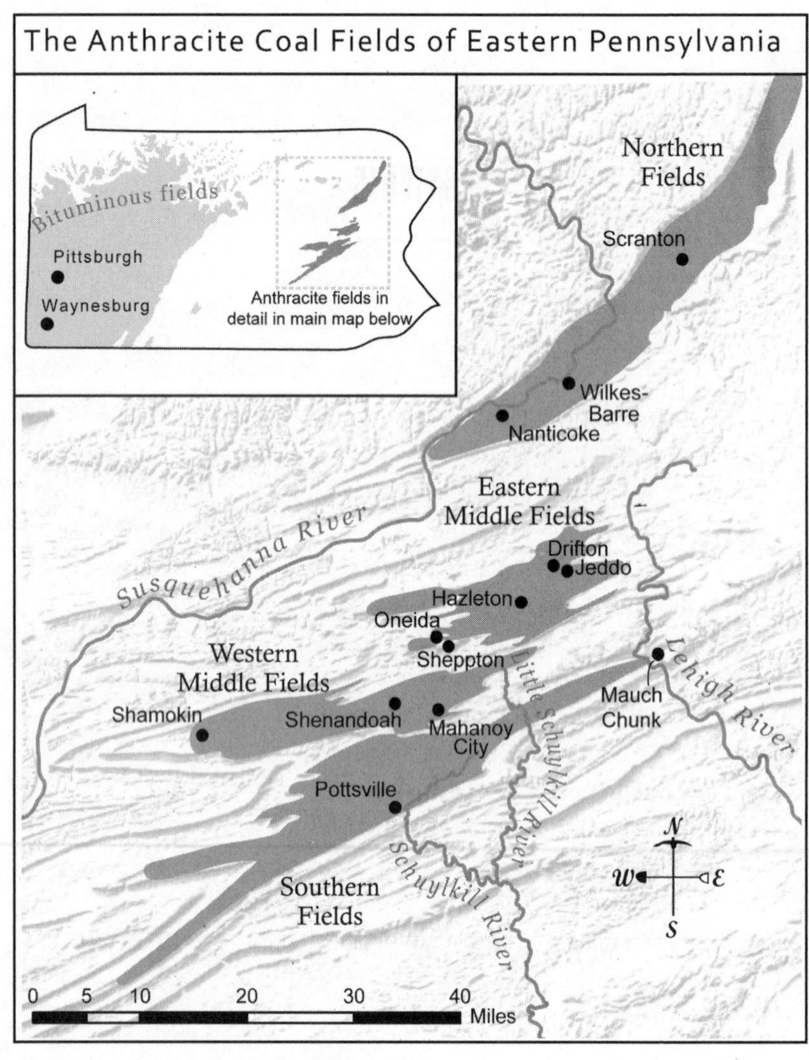

The Anthracite Coal Fields of Eastern Pennsylvania
Bituminous fields
Pittsburgh
Waynesburg
Anthracite fields in detail in main map below
Northern Fields
Scranton
Wilkes-Barre
Nanticoke
Eastern Middle Fields
Drifton
Jeddo
Hazleton
Oneida
Sheppton
Western Middle Fields
Shamokin
Shenandoah
Mahanoy City
Mauch Chunk
Pottsville
Southern Fields
Susquehanna River
Little Schuylkill River
Schuylkill River
Lehigh River
N
W
E
S
0
5
10
20
30
40
Miles

PREFACE

Nearly 150,000 hard-rock coal miners walked out of the eastern Pennsylvania coal mines on May 12, 1902, launching a strike that would remake the labor movement in the United States, reshape the relationship of the federal government to labor and industry, and launch a period of Progressive Era reforms that would give rise to the institution of police as we know it. They did it without their union leaders' support and with the entire Pennsylvania National Guard mobilized against them. The coal companies, owned by the wealthiest men in the country, built an army of private police to starve them back to the mines. They went on strike anyway, and over the course of five dramatic months, at the dawn of the twentieth century, their struggle electrified working people everywhere.

Though amazing histories and studies of the coalcrackers' lives and struggles have been written, no story of this strike has ever been told from the perspective of the miners who launched it. Instead the story of the strike has been told from the perspective of the coal-company presidents, sheriffs, military generals, political reformists, and labor leaders. Every history of the story has been told from their perspective, in their voice. It's been told as the story of the saving of American capitalism by farsighted industrialists whose compromises stabilized industrial production and made America great. It's been told as the story of pragmatic union leaders, newly committed to law and order, who brought the labor movement into the mainstream by rescuing working people from their violent and radical tendencies. It's been told as the story of the remaking of American politics by reform-minded politicians who carved out a conservative path for working people, one we still tread today. As a result, if we know the strike at all, we know it as the story of a great victory won on behalf of working people told from the perspective of those who despised the coal miners.

This book tells the story of that long-forgotten strike once again but, for the first time, from the perspective and, more importantly, through and with the words of the miners, whose voices I unearthed in the archive. The words of thousands of mine workers, their widows, and their children, like a buried parade of discarded stories, fill the archives with harrowing tales of migrations across oceans, of dangerous work done deep underground, of being blacklisted from jobs and evicted from homes, of surviving one hostile place after another. Widows whose names no one bothered to record told of lives lived in the aftermath of husband's or sons' violent deaths. Little breaker boys who looked as if they'd been dug out of the earth told stories that read like nightmares. Anonymous scribes at fateful union meetings captured in their notes all the turmoil and terror of people who knew they were being used up and who were fighting to keep from being cast aside.

To finally read their words is to enter their world. Throughout the book, I use italics instead of quotation marks to indicate the exact speech of actual people as it was recorded when spoken, or to indicate the exact written words of published material from a newspaper, book, article, or document from the archive. All references, including citations for italicized phrases, can be found at the end of the book.

The use of italics is not intended as a gimmick. The point is not to speak for the miners or to bring the dead back to life, but to find a narrative style of historical writing that best captures their world, one full of hope and upheaval during a strike, a world-historical event, which exploded like a thunderbolt in their lives. Their voices have occasionally surfaced in other stories written about the strike, but only to briefly flicker by before disappearing once again. By rendering their words in italics, like a brand burned on the page, they stake a claim to this version of their story. For once, they occupy their own history. This is an open style of historical writing that refuses to see the past as settled, or as a record of progress, or as a cautionary tale. The method I adopt for this book is a method for writing a miners' history, a story told by people who worked hard, were paid little, and died young. A story told by people whose voices didn't matter, whose past was considered a problem, whose dreams were ignored, and whose futures every American institution mobilized to thwart.

I recreate scenes and brief moments in their lives by giving over the text to their words, by adopting their language, and by merging my words with theirs. Some may object to this method and call it one-sided or partisan. So be it. I have the same objection to all the histories that ignored them. By leaving their voices buried in the archives, we've lost the real significance of the strike. If the job of the historian is to capture the past in all its complexity and meaning, then no history of the great anthracite strike of 1902 has ever been written. What we call history is not what the miners called their present, and our present is not the future the miners fought for. They had something else in mind.

INTRODUCTION

DIG ANOTHER GRAVE

On the day they abolished the police, June 17, 1935, Michael Musmanno, fresh from lawyering Sacco and Vanzetti, climbed onto a Waynesburg, Pennsylvania, stage to deliver a mock eulogy and got hit in the head with a brick. He wasn't even mad. It was a glancing blow. And besides, it wasn't like the kid who threw it had malice in his heart, other than for the police. It was an errant toss. The target had been the effigy of a cop's *corpse* swinging from a gallows attached to the top of a car in front of the stage. Musmanno, the Pennsylvania state legislator whose *bill killed the system* of private industrial police, or at least tried to, shook off the blow and stayed on script. *This encourages us that we can win another fight*, he said to the roar of fifteen thousand people cheering the striking coal miners as they cut the effigy down and stuffed it into a pine box. *In the not too-distant future*, said Musmanno, speaking directly to the coffin, *we will dig another grave for your murderous cousin, the company-paid deputy sheriff.*

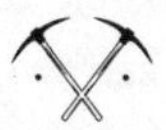

Six years earlier, on a cold February night in 1929, Harold Watts and Frank Slapikas, two drunk cops looking for a place to keep drinking, saw a light on at Blussick's boardinghouse in Santi-

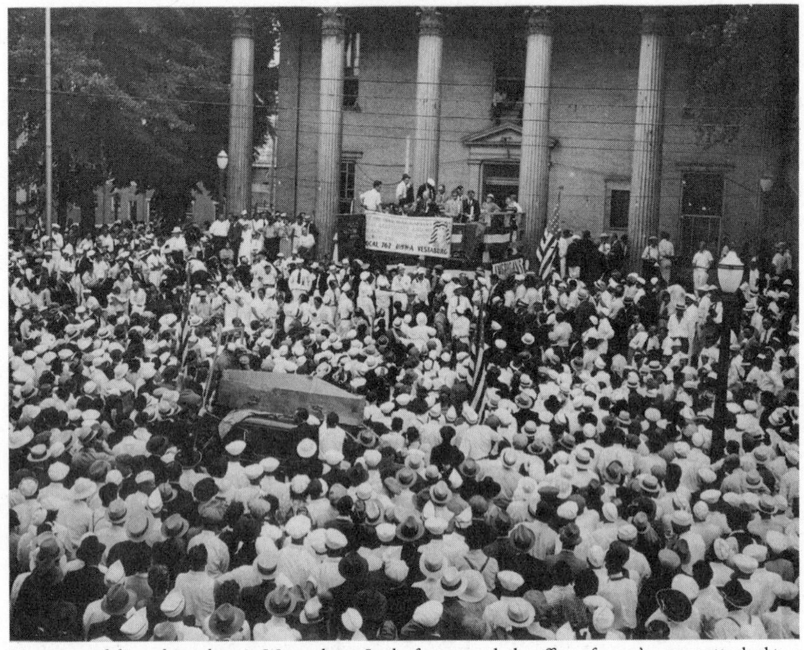

Musmanno delivers his eulogy in Waynesburg. In the foreground, the effigy of a cop's corpse attached to a pine box makes its way through the crowd. Courtesy: Duquesne University Archives.

ago, Pennsylvania. They stopped to see if John Higgins, an ex-cop and Blussick boarder, was home. Higgins invited them in, and the men sat in the front room drinking whiskey from a pint that Watts pulled from his coat.

In the kitchen, two rooms away, Mrs. Blussick sat with her son-in-law, the Polish miner John Borcoski, still wearing his blue work overalls from a shift at his job at the Pittsburgh Coal Company's Montour Mine #9. Back in the front room, there was another knock at the door. Eddie Blussick, another Montour miner and a son of Mrs. Blussick, arrived with two other union miners. He was surprised to see two cops in his mother's boardinghouse. With Blussick standing over him, Watts lit a Lucky Strike, and as he took his first drag, one of the miners with Blussick said, The only man *who'd smoke a Lucky is a klansman.* The argument that followed echoed through the house and brought

Patsy Caruso, another boarder, into the room. Caruso stepped between the arguing men and gave Watts a dirty look. *I thought you were a better man*, she said to him. When Watts pushed her away, Higgins ordered everyone out. They argued as they went, and their yelling alarmed Mrs. Blussick, who asked Borcoski to tell them to keep it down. Sure, he said, and he walked through the front room past Caruso and out the front door. In the dark, pointing his miner's lamp, he saw the men arguing in a cop car parked in the driveway. He shined the light into the car as he walked toward them. Watts jumped out of the car when he arrived and pistol-whipped him with his handgun, knocking him to the ground. Borcoski scrambled to his feet and stumbled back to the house, leaving a trail of blood. Caruso came running out when she heard the commotion and watched Watts chase Borcoski back to the house. She yelled at Watts to leave Borcoski alone, then ducked and ran when Watts pointed his revolver at her. Watts caught up to Borcoski at the door, and the two men crashed into the front room. Slapikas came barreling in after them. He grabbed Higgins and held him back while Watts beat Borcoski in the head with a three-fingered knuckler, opening a deeper cut that covered the carpet with blood. Borcoski managed to wrestle himself free from Watts and run from the room. While Slapikas hauled Higgins to the car, Watts chased after Borcoski and caught up to him in the front yard of the house, where he tackled him to the ground, cuffed his arms behind his back, and dragged him to the cop car. With their prisoners in the back seat, Watts and Slapikas drove wildly back to the Pittsburgh Coal Company's police barracks in Imperial.

When they arrived at the station, Watts dropped Borcoski in a heap on the barracks floor and then began hitting Higgins in the head with a club, knocking him unconscious. Slapikas hauled Higgins into another room and shackled him to a prisoner rail. The Glenfield constable Ross Shafer was in the barracks when the men arrived but left as soon as the beating began.

It was none of my business, he would say later. Watts called for a doctor but not out of any concern for Borcoski or Higgins. When Dr. J. M. Patterson arrived, Watts said he'd been stabbed in the back, but all the doctor saw was a scratch. *When I arrived,* Patterson would say later, *Borcoski was lying on the floor against the wall. He was covered in blood.* While Borcoski moaned in pain, the doctor cut blood-soaked hair from open wounds and covered them in bandages. *He'd been hit with a blunt instrument of some sort,* guessed Patterson. *There were various ribs broken.*

Walter Lyster, the lieutenant in charge of the Imperial barracks, showed up at three o'clock in the morning and found Borcoski lying in his own blood. He turned smiling to Watts and Slapikas, like a child on Christmas morning. *I feel like having a workout.* He disappeared into the locker room and returned wearing work pants and a gray flannel shirt and holding a four-foot leather strap, which he used to beat Borcoski on the head. The doctor stood and watched the beating, intervening only to reapply bandages dislodged by Lyster's blows. *I saw him kick Borcoski violently in the side,* said the doctor. *Lyster was trying to get some information from Borcoski, but Borcoski didn't know what it was.* By four o'clock in the morning Borcoski's face *had turned blue* and his nose had been *flattened* by the blows. The doctor announced he had to leave and suggested the cops lay off the poor guy. Borcoski put a hand on the wall and pulled himself to his knees, breathing heavily and whipping blood from his eyes. Lyster waited until the doctor had left and then came at Borcoski with a fireplace poker, hitting him in the head so many times and with such force that it bent in half. When he stopped to bend it back straight, Watts jumped in and poured boiling water on Borcoski and then jumped on his chest until he heard the sound of bones breaking.

When the doctor returned an hour or so later, he walked in to find Watts jumping on Borcoski's chest, Slapikas kicking him in the head, and Lyster swinging his half-bent poker, the three of them *delighting in the impact of the whip, club and fist upon bare flesh,* stopping only when they grew tired. When they did, the doctor replaced Borcoski's bandages and added new ones to cover new wounds, which Lyster pulled off when the doctor left. He waterboarded Borcoski while Watts and Slapikas kicked him in the head and body. Higgins would say later he heard ribs snap from the other room and the sound of Borcoski desperately pleading with the cops that he couldn't breathe.

When it was over, and Borcoski lay corpselike on the floor, the three cops cleaned blood from their hands and faces, changed clothes, and woke Shafer, who had slept through the beating in another room. They ordered him to drive Borcoski to Sewickley hospital. I had to do what they said, Shafer explained later. *I was afraid of them.* The doctor pronounced Borcoski dead on arrival, attributing his death *to a mass of lacerations and bruises.* His *rib structure was fractured, his lungs punctured, his nose broken, hands swollen twice their size.*

When Borcoski didn't return home, his wife, Sofia, went out looking for him. She stopped first at her mother's, who told her the cops had taken him to Imperial the night before. She went to the barracks, but Watts and Slapikas had already left. *I want my man*, she said to the cop on duty, but he slammed the door in her face. She went around back and knocked until another cop answered.

What did you do with my husband?
We sent him to the hospital.
Why did you do that?
He was sick.
He wasn't sick when you got him.
Well, he cut one of our men.

She went to the hospital, but the nurse wouldn't let her see her husband. He's dead, she was told. Borcoski's sister and brother stopped at the barracks after Sofia and found the cops still mopping up blood from the floor and wiping it from the walls.

Sofia buried her husband in the St. Columbkill Catholic cemetery three days later. No eulogy was offered, she just stood by the grave in stunned silence holding her four children while five hundred miners huddled around them. After the burial, as she walked from the cemetery, a reporter asked her if she had any comment, and all she could say was, *life isn't safe.*

On the day of the funeral, the *Pittsburgh Post-Gazette* ran a series of stories about Lyster and Watts. It wasn't the first time either of them had killed a miner or beaten a man to death. When Lyster worked as a state cop, he'd killed a striking miner with an axe during the uprising at Lilly in 1923. Watts had murdered a Black man named M. C. Watkins in 1927 after he'd come to the defense of a woman Watts had been beating. A Pittsburgh jury acquitted Lyster, Watts, and Slapikas of murder, but the judge threw it out and called the jurors incompetent and *without moral stamina.* Prosecutors recharged them with involuntary manslaughter, but Slapikas was acquitted again. Watts and Lyster were convicted and sentenced to twenty-two months on a work detail.

The Pittsburgh Coal Company released a statement before the trial calling Lyster a fine officer and its private army of Coal and Iron Police *a body of men trained and experienced in work of this kind of whom we are justly proud.* The millionaire Mellon family, which owned the Pittsburgh Coal Company and controlled a coalfield twice the size of Rhode Island, spent one million dollars a year on cops to patrol a labor force of nine thousand miners who toiled for wages as low as a dollar a day. Musmanno sued the Mellons on Sofia's behalf. She eventually won a $13,000 settlement, which she used as a down payment on a farm that she and her husband had always dreamed of buying, but she couldn't make a go of it alone and lost it to the bank a year later.

Musmanno blamed the shocking torture and murder of John Borcoski on Pennsylvania's system of private policing. The 1865 statute that created the Coal and Iron Police gave railroad companies, coal collieries, furnaces, and rolling mills the legal right to create armies of strikebreaking police vested with *all the powers of policemen of the city of Philadelphia.* Private cops with official state commissions had the legal authority to patrol beyond the boundaries of coal-company property. The statute made it clear: cops work on behalf of the coal companies, *but their powers are more general.* Their discretion to use violence under color of law in the interest of their employers was nearly unlimited.

Musmanno led the crusade to abolish the whole system. As a young legislator, he filed a bill to put an end to the Coal and Iron Police, but the only result was a name change. The Coal and Iron Police would now be called industrial police. Otherwise, there would be no difference. The same system of policing, using the same arbitrary violence against working people, producing the same industrial order, under a new name. Musmanno, undeterred, kept up his campaign. He gave speeches and wrote editorials describing the Coal and Iron Police as a unique kind of evil. Its birth in the late nineteenth century transformed policing from the ad hoc, vigilante violence of settlers to the formal and official vigilantism of company-paid thugs operating under color of law.

Musmanno's focus was on Pennsylvania's Coal and Iron Police, but the more he dug, the more private police he unearthed. Nearly every state developed systems of private policing in the late nineteenth century, whether by statute or common practice. Wherever you found a laboring poor, you found private cops on patrol, in every industry. Railroad police, roadhouse police, eatery police, quarry police, electric police, merchant police, steamboat police, coal and iron police, constables paid by subscription, sheriff's deputies sworn in for strikebreaking duty, night watchmen and private guards holding public commissions. In most states, the origins of private and semi-private policing could be found in the wake of the nationwide railroad strike of 1877, which had *revealed the power of a unified working class.* It was no longer enough to recruit private cops in times of strike, concluded the railroad presidents and industrialists. They called for a permanent system of policing to be established town by town, industry by industry. Most operated like the cavalry or a military platoon, others like a municipal police department, some like the old slave patrols. Others were extensions of the militias of the Indian Wars. Some cities gave police commissions to people who defined their bailiwick based on the distribution of residents or merchants willing to pay them. Nearly all municipal constables were paid, in part or full, by the fines they collected from the people they arrested. Railroad police operated in North Carolina, Rhode Island, and North Dakota. West Virginia and Kentucky allowed collieries to join railroads in building private police forces, same as Pennsylvania. Steamboat police operated in California, New York, and Rhode Island. County sheriffs in Virginia, South Carolina, Iowa, South Dakota, and Minnesota appointed special police deputies paid by the companies that requested them. Connecticut, Ohio, Georgia, and Alabama allowed private corporations to petition the governor to cede police powers to private corporations *under certain contingencies or extraordinary circumstances.* Illinois prohibited *so-called industrial police* but allowed business owners in cities and villages to create their own *merchant police* who operated with official commissions. Maine, Indiana, and Washington let cities outsource policing to private companies.

The only reason Pennsylvania had more, and more notorious, private police was because of the coal buried in the ground, particularly the hard anthracite coal found only in the earth below five small counties in eastern Pennsylvania. Anthracite burned hotter and longer than the softer, bituminous or lignite coal found everywhere else. It produced less smoke and soot, making it an ideal fuel for factories and mills in cities and as a replacement for wood, charcoal, and imported soft coal for domestic fuel. By 1855, Pennsylvania's anthracite fired nearly every blast furnace in the United States, powered every steamship that crossed the Atlantic, fired every boiler in every factory and hotel, and heated every home and hearth up and down the Eastern Seaboard. Admirals declared its availability a matter of national security. Business professors claimed it kickstarted the iron industry and made industrial development possible, which in turn created a new, industrial working class and gave rise to a managerial class.

In June of 1931, when the initial legislation to abolish industrial police failed, Pennsylvania governor Gifford Pinchot revoked all industrial police commissions, but this made no difference at all. The coal companies just pivoted to the county sheriffs, who commissioned private deputies on their behalf. Now the cops were called private deputies, roving detectives, special policemen. The same system of policing, the same arbitrary violence against working people, under a new name. During a 1934 strike, hundreds of private deputy sheriffs broke up picket lines with *tear gas, buckshot and machine guns.* Private cops put sixty bullets in one striker's leg and seventy-five into another. They fired a bullet into one miner's face and seven into another's. There were so many bullet holes and so much buckshot in the body of one miner that the coroner refused to guess how many times he'd been shot. Private deputies killed one picketing striker just for standing in the road. They shot into a crowd of children in Broughton. A woman lying in bed got hit in the hip by a cop's rifleshot and never walked again. It seemed like every effort to fix or abolish private police only intensified the violence of police, like a beast gone berserk.

The vicious and brutal years that followed the murder of John Borcoski sharpened Musmanno's criticisms of private police. *They have been guilty of every crime on the calendar. They have acted as spies and provocateurs. They have used their clubs, blackjacks, revolvers on miners. They have wounded, maimed, and killed innocent people. They have forced their lecherous attention on girls and women without protection. They have stirred up trouble and strife just to satisfy their sadistic urge to swing clubs on human heads. Many have been recruited from gunmen, thugs, and criminals. They have fired on schoolhouses and school children. They have tortured and used every form of hellish third degree on unfortunate prisoners. They shot dogs. They jumped their horses over babies.*

Musmanno hated the Coal and Iron Police, but he was no abolitionist. While he decried industrial policing as *a sale of police power by the State*, he praised police in general. The problem wasn't police, he always said, the problem was private police on the payroll of the coal companies. What we need, he argued, were permanent agencies of public police staffed by professional officers. He found support for the argument among Progressive Era reformers who saw Pennsylvania's system of private policing as an aberration. It was antidemocratic, they complained. The sale of policing to the private sector cheapened *the sovereignty of the Commonwealth.* But the police, they argued, were essential to a stable, industrial order. We will make police accountable to the public, they promised. We will organize police into official departments where they will no longer serve the interests of private corporations.

Most establishment histories of the police trace its modern origins to this moment, crediting Progressive-Era reformers like Musmanno for creating the institution of police as we know it. It was through their Progressive reforms, the story goes, that the Coal and Iron Police were abolished, and goons were transformed into public servants, gunmen into professional police, and all were held accountable by law. But this is the fairytale story we tell about the police. Borcoski's murder in 1929 and

Musmanno's reforms in the mid-1930s didn't abolish industrial policing and don't mark the moment that modern police were created. The birth of the institution of police came decades earlier, as part of a backlash that followed the rise of the United Mine Workers of America.

If there was one moment or one event that marked the birth of the police, it was the great Anthracite Coal Strike of 1902, when 150,000 union miners of the recently formed United Mine Workers of America laid down their tools and walked out of the mines. Their labor leaders opposed the strike, but the miners were desperate for a different world. Their working lives had been defined by mine collapses and explosions that killed so many of them, and so consistently, that the state of Pennsylvania measured mine productivity in tons of coal produced per number of miners killed. And yet, despite decades of efforts, no miners' union had ever found a way to defeat the coal companies and their strikebreakers. Solidarity seemed forever beyond their grasp. Mine owners used blacklists to keep the miners divided by race and ethnicity. Conservative labor leaders, time and time again, argued for patience and compromise despite lethal working conditions and low wages. They convinced the miners to compromise, or sold them out, or were bought off themselves. When the strike started, the coal companies, as they always did, called the miners terrorists, played up the so-called threat of unassimilable immigrant miners, and sent more than five thousand Coal and Iron Police into the five anthracite-producing counties. County sheriffs augmented these forces with private armies of their own. The Pennsylvania governor sent ten thousand National Guard troops into the coalfields to force them back to work. Reporters covered every moment of the five-month strike, plastering their front pages with stories of intimidation and police murder, of constant clashes between strikers and private police, of defiant mine communities fighting police and refusing to compromise.

Despite their cautious leaders and everything that divided them, the miners somehow built a vast and unyielding solidarity. Almost overnight, the union became a united, multiethnic force ten times the size of the combined agencies of all the private police. Nearly every day during the strike, thousands of miners and their supporters marched through mine patches and coal towns behind fife and drum corps, shouting at the cops and intimidating the scabs. They hung effigies of scabs from telegraph poles. Their children threw rocks at cops. The police fired pistols and rifles into crowds. Women boycotted the stores that sold to scabs. Priests refused to give replacement workers last rites. Magazines published moving stories about the plight of miserable, debt-bound miners and their families. Donations flooded into the union strike fund. Constables, deputies, and even some National Guard troops feared for their lives. They refused to serve as strikebreakers and some even openly supported the union. Suddenly, an entire social order based on private property and wage labor teetered on the brink.

The coal companies raised the alarm. If we let the miners win the fight, these rough working people will seize control of the coal industry and dictate the path of future industrial development in the United States and beyond. There will be no wage, no private property, no role for the businessman to play in a world run by the working class. They demanded federal troops, more state troops, more sheriff's deputies, but none of it worked. The Coal and Iron Police proved unable to starve the miners back to the mines. The militia collapsed in the face of enormous crowds of determined strikers. The coal presidents begged the federal government for help, but President Teddy Roosevelt refused to send federal troops. This is a fight for the future of America, they declared, and we're losing.

In the middle of a strike that looked lost, a consortium of coal companies announced the creation of a new strikebreaking strategy. They abandoned their usual tactics and instead converted the coalfields into a living laboratory for the development of what became a new kind of police. Their innovations remain with us today. They recruited military veterans with strikebreaking experience and created the first special tactics and weapons unit in the United States. They combined dozens of small, ad hoc, private police forces into one large, multicounty police force. When the strike ended, the state of Pennsylvania created the first department of state police in the United States, designed by the men who fought the miners, and modeled on the version of policing they used to defeat the strike. This new version of the police was a permanent, professional agency, but the coal companies didn't create this new version of the police for its democratic potential or its ability to hold police accountable. *We have the state constabulary law,* wrote a mine president to his Wall Street financier, *which affords more protection to our industry than any other class of industry, and as we know has saved us money.* The police mandate is order, and the order the coal companies had in mind was one capable of defending private property, imposing wage labor, and guarding their private interests. By the time Musmanno eulogized industrial policing on that Waynesburg, Pennsylvania, stage in 1935, his promise of a new era of public and professional police had already been proven wrong, and by thirty years.

This book tells the story of the strike of 1902 and the birth of the institution of police. It's a story of the rough and rowdy miners of eastern Pennsylvania and the fight they waged at the dawn of the twentieth century, a fight Samuel Gompers called *the most important single incident in the labor movement,* a strike John Mitchell, the young president of the United Mine Workers, called *the fiercest struggle in which we have yet engaged*. It's the story of 150,000 of the lowest paid laborers in the country who worked the most dangerous job in the world and who emerged from deep inside the earth to challenge the power of the wealthiest men on the planet. The strike of 1902 nearly destroyed an industrial order that for over a hundred years had been based on the violent company control of the mines and of every facet of the miners' lives. For a fleeting moment, the strike brought industry after industry to its knees, giving the miners a brief glimpse of a working life free from the suffocating wages of the mine bosses and out from under the iron heel of the Coal and Iron Police. A different world came into focus, one organized to meet the needs of those with the least, not one dominated by those who'd stolen the most. A moment ruthlessly beaten back by a new kind of police, one built by the mine owners from the ashes of the old. This is the story of that long fight and brief victory and of the new police unleashed to pacify the miners, destroy their union, and force them back into the ground. This is the story of those miners, that great struggle, and the birth of the institution of police as we know it.

CHAPTER ONE

A GOOD PRACTICAL MINER

Dig deep and find rivers of rock buried below ridges and valleys, rich deposits of a coastal plain's bogs and rias gone into hiding. Pierce these underground forests of ferns and fast growing trees with shafts that drop from the surface like elevators, or drifts that start low in the basin and then rise up through ridges, or slopes that invade outcroppings and then chase the coal deep into the earth. At the mouth, descend by foot, rail, or wooden box. Arrive at the bottom to the branching gangways and muleways that lead to where the miners work, the tomblike chambers that float inside the earth, like submerged piers bobbing on petrified floes of rock. In these breasts, in the crosscut of a vein, find the face of the coal. Hold your candle up, bring light to the dark, take stock of the air. Best if it's a strong, steady flame, which tells you the black damp is weak. Pay heed to a flickering flame, for your life is out of your hands. Attach the oil lamp to your cap and inspect the timbers and weight-bearing pillars of coal that hold up the earth. Find signs of their future collapse in the scattered slivers of wood and flakes of coal that collect on the floor, shed from the pillars by the squeeze of the earth's weight. Tear out a tin of Frishmuth and share a smoke with your *butty* before bringing your attention back to the face of the coal, the long wall you're paid to push into the earth. Run your hand along its surface, tracing the outline of whole trees and the run of resin that once traveled their length, thermochemical timeprints of the stored energy of another earth's sun, as infinite as the past. No end in sight.

Above you hangs a series of strings from the roof that mark the outer limits and direction of the vein you will drive. Suspended between those strings and stretching from the face back to the gangway hang the brattices that move the bad air out and make a path for the good air to flow in. Know that everything is alive, always in a state of becoming, never finished. At the face, a vein looks like a solid wall, but inside the earth, nothing is what it appears. A vein is not a thing, it is a chase, and it has the jump on you, folding and twisting as it races away into earth, thickening, splitting in half, reforming. Some pitch nearly perpendicular to the surface and then erupt into outcropped ridges. Other veins dive under rivers and boroughs, racing along a horizontal path. Some start thick then pinch to nothing. Some glisten shiny black then turn bony and sulfurous.

This is anthracite, the eastern Pennsylvania hard coal that refuses to be dug with shovels like the soft lignite that burns with a black smoke and leaves a thick soot. It resists the pickaxe and won't be easily hacked at by hand as in the bituminous mines everywhere else. It requires patience and as many kegs of black powder as you can afford. Powder is a low explosive, which works only when buried in the rock, which is true of the miners too. It takes skill and hard labor to set the earth on fire. Start by placing the chiseled bit of your long miners' drill to the face of the coal. Lean into the iron and crank the drill, listening with your body for the sound and strain of rock giving way. When the hole is as deep as you are tall, draw out the drill and scrape the rock clean. It's impossible to say in general how any of this should be done. There is no standard rule or guide, no single way to approach the face, no set number of holes to drill, nothing knowable for certain. *It is a piece of work that can never be learned.*

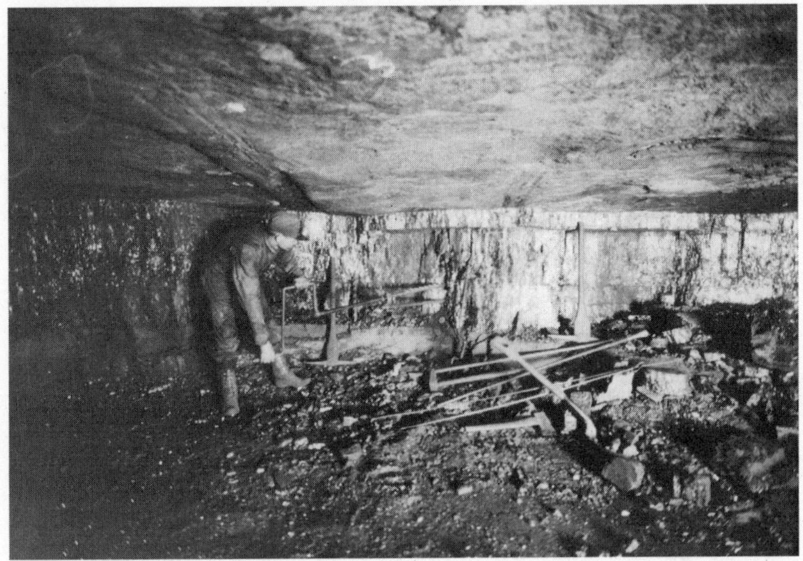

Drilling into the face of the coal. Courtesy: Indiana University of Pennsylvania Special Collections and University Archive.

But learn it quickly because your life depends on it. A poorly placed hole might blow out part of a wall, leaving a ledge of coal. You'll find yourself lying on your back in water, working at the underside of a cantilevered bench that waits to crush you. Some holes hit sulfur balls harder than any rock; others drill easy. Some holes drill dry until *water gushes out of them.* Some holes fill the breast with pockets of methane, what the good practical miner calls firedamp, a living, malevolent gas that hides in your lungs and hopes for a spark. A good practical miner learns how to avoid this, learns where to hang the brattices to keep the air moving, learns how to drill around the sulfur, learns how to blast a wall free without weakening the props, learns how to fire a wet shot without wasting powder, *but an inexperienced man loses powder there. He does not know how to fire wet shots, and that deters his work, as well as making his expenses heavy.* Tell an inexperienced man to leave a place like that. *Put a practical man in his place*, before it's too late.

After the holes are drilled in the right places and at the right depths, slide your black powder cartridges into the holes, tamping them tight, half a dozen per hole. These are the explosive cartridges you make yourself. A careful scoop of powder into cardboard paper wrapped into the shape of a bullet as big as your forearm. Once tamped into place, slide your long, miners' needle into each hole, carefully piercing the cartridges. Use caution. Drilling a hole in rock and then filling it with black powder is, as the blinded Welshman John Price learned, like building your own cannon, loading it with gunpowder, and then staring into the barrel while lighting the fuse. *I went to pull the pin out, and I happened to shove the needle through the powder, and it struck fire to the sulphur.* The spark *exploded the powder, and I was right in front of the hole.* The blast took Price's eye and mangled his hand.

Avoid Price's fate by using a copper miners' needle, which doesn't spark, but good luck affording that, what with all the deductions and supplies the bosses take from your wages—the money for the doctor, the portion for your rent, the wages withheld for food bought at the company store. It adds up and never ends. The two picks and two drills for $1.25 each. An eight-pound pick at $0.80. Two shovels for $1.20. A $0.90 hammer. A $0.75 axe and a saw for $2.75. Don't enter a mine without a length of pulley chain; something around forty feet is enough, and that's at least $5, though likely more. The blacksmith fee gets deducted directly, but you won't get what you pay for. The blacksmith will refuse you when you ask for a sharpen. The bosses have him doing a thousand other things. So, swallow the $0.13 a month you pay for blacksmithing that you don't get, and spend another $0.10 a month on a file so you can sharpen your tools yourself. Some miners now use the automatic Legrand drill instead of the manual one, but those cost $12, and the rock eats a $0.50 cent bit every month. Even changing the bit costs money. Only the contract miners with teams of laborers and sweetheart deals with the bosses use that. The squibs that spark the powder cost $0.25 each. Buy two boxes a month, if not more. Buy three blasting barrels a month, at $0.06 a foot. You'll need a pound of cotton each month. You'll burn a $0.30 gallon of oil in the lamp attached to your cap for every ten or so feet you dig into the earth. Buy more than one. You'll need a toolbox to hold it all, and that'll cost you $1.50 easy. Count yourself lucky when your paycheck isn't an empty envelope, common enough there's even name for it: a bobtail check.

John Price saved money by using an iron needle instead of a copper one, and it cost him in the end. If you use the iron needle, remove it with the same patience you use with the bosses. Then slide a fused squib into each pierced cartridge. Gather up the fuses that fall like tails from the face. Tie them together into one long fuse. Before lighting it, take fistfuls of mud and dirt and pack each hole closed. The mud traps the blast in the rock, turning the face into a wall of guns that you have loaded yourself. Push from your mind that you have made the earth into a firing squad that you stand before like some poor man condemned to labor for a dollar a day in the making of his own death.

Set the earth on fire by lighting the tangled fuses with the burning oil lamp on your cap. Holler a warning and take cover. Say a prayer the fuse won't fizzle. *A man may go to look after his fuse thinking it has gone out, and it explodes.* The coal will be *driven into the face or into the head, through the skull often, into the chest or into the abdomen, destroying life at once.* Or maybe, like the Scranton miner David Davis, your fuse will start but then half-stop. Davis lit two holes that he'd fused together and then took cover, but when he returned to the breast after the explosion, he found that one of the fuses had fizzled and paused. *I squeezed the fuse to squeeze the dead fire out and when the first one went out, I went back to light the fuse the second time and when I got hold of the fuse, away she went. My left eye was blown out clean, and my right eye was blown out on my forehead, and that went out in the hospital. My left ear was not blown off, it was cut off, it was hanging. The blast left a big hole in my chest. I make my living now selling little supplies for the miners such as oil and squibs, and so forth.*

Ask a mine inspector what causes the miners' deaths. He'll say carelessness and inexperience, but don't believe him. Was it carelessness and inexperience that doomed the Irishman Neal McDonigle? It's true, despite forty years mining coal, he fired a shot in a breast fouled with firedamp, but what could he do? *I told the boss one day, I says: The air is so bad. I will quit working. He says: If you do, you will get no cars for the other breast you have. I thought I had better work on the same as the rest, because I knowed if I did not, he would keep the cars from the other breast, and I would make nothing.* Having no choice, he fired a shot *which ignited* a fireball that *blowed us up, me and my butty. My butty lived four days afterwards.* McDonigle spent six months lying in a special bed made of water.

Even if your shot doesn't engulf the mine in fire, the blast will fill the air with powder smoke so heavy you can *weigh it on scales by the pound. It is something so thick you cannot go through, or it would cut you blind.* Wait for the brattices to clear the smoke. If the company refuses the expense of the brattices, expect to work in thick smoke for hours. What choice do you have? When the smoke clears, find the floor littered with a kaleidoscope of spores that once floated in pale, carboniferous skies, and now, hundreds of millions of years later, pockmarks the skin of the coal you've blown free from the face. Before you finish the face, take the heel end of your pick and tap the roof, sounding the top coal, listening for the absence of sound that foretells a rockfall. If you hear what cannot be heard, summon the timberboss for more timber props to hold up the earth. A good mine will send company miners down to your breast and they will shore up your roof with the timbers they drag into the earth with them. More likely you'll be made to do it yourself and won't get any allowance pay for it.

After shoring up the roof, turn your attention back to the blown-out face, where you will find the outline of ancient leaves that survived eras and ages of heat and pressure debossing the surface of half-freed rocks still clinging to the earth. Use your axe or heavy pick to finish the job, taking care to avoid the explosions of razor-sharp slivers and dagger-like shards of coal that erupt with each swing into rock. When you have freed all the coal that can be freed, draw your gob rake across the floor, separating dirt and slate from coal. Tell your laborer, if you have one, or your butty, if you work two-handed, to drag the buggy in from the gangway, so you can shovel up the coal. If you're lucky, you get sixty cents a car for each miners' ton of coal you send up the shaft, maybe more, depends on the vein. This isn't a wage, so don't mistake it as some kind of agreed-to thing. The bosses say that a thousand pounds of every ton that a miner digs from the earth is nothing but waste—bony slate, they'll call it, dirt laced with coal, they'll insist. They account for this so-called waste by paying on the basis of the miners' ton, which is somewhere between 2,800 and 3,300 pounds and is measured by the quick glance of a docking boss up at the top of the breaker. Say you make a deal for a breast with a foreman on the miners' ton basis of sixty cents a car. The car itself provides a rough measure of a miners' ton, even though the cars are not a uniform size and *are always getting larger.* You'll be required to fill the car and then top it off six inches above water height. That's a miner's ton, no matter the size of the car or how much everything weighs.

The bosses claim the topping is necessary to account for the settling that happens as the coal makes its trip from the breast to the shaft and up into the breaker where the coal is sorted. They say the miners load the cars light, *cribbing*, they call it, the strategy of underfilling the cars with *the coal in a manner that permitted a maximum amount of space between lumps.* You'll be made to fill it high before the teenage muledriver will take it from your breast to the shaft bottom. It will be hoisted out of the mine and sent to the top of the breaker, where a docking boss waits. In the seconds it takes for the car to dump its load, he will measure your coal with a glance, docking you for loading light or for loading dirty coal. There's no way to protect yourself from this. It's a long trip from the bottom of the mine to the top of the breaker. Along the way, the coal will settle, no matter how high you stack it. Some will get tossed out when the engineer hoists it up the shaft. The only way to keep the coal above water height is by stacking it like an overfilled ice cream cone. But even if you load the car tight and it arrives at the breaker six inches above the water height, the boss will dock you anyway. Too much dirt, he'll claim, even though the miners' ton accounts for it. Too much slate, he'll say, even though what looks like slate is often *a shell of slate covering coal.* Whenever the miners win a wage increase, this is how the docking bosses take it back. *No matter how heavy we loaded our cars, we would be docked anyhow.* You and your butty will load four cars in a day if you're lucky. Count on the docking boss taking *a half or maybe three-quarters of what you deliver.* You make your wage by mining coal, and the bosses make their money by mining you.

The mining of anthracite, which is found only in the earth below eastern Pennsylvania's river valleys and folded ridges, turns the earth inside out and reshapes the surface. Rivers that once cut through valleys now follow shafts deep into the earth. Creeks that once fed rivers now run black from mine waste and the runoff of clearcut forests. In the early years, before the railroads, anthracite traveled to market by arks launched by oarsmen into rivers flooded by spring freshets. Half or more of the cargo was lost when the arks stoved into the rocks. Later came the rafts that floated down hand-dug canals pulled by teams of horses laboring along parallel tow paths. Now, in 1902, it is delivered by rail to tidewater, sold by brokers, burned in blast furnaces and steam engines, and used to fuel an armada of steamships fired across oceans from an Eastern seaboard's yet unburied coastal plain.

It's a magical thing—a rock that burns. When it catches fire, it burns hotter and longer than wood or soft coal and seems liberated from smoke and soot, as if all of earth's past and present suddenly appeared in material form, transforming the present into the future. The engineers of progress welcomed it all. Look at this new working class it made. Look at this new industrial managerial class it conjured. They charted a path to a future by releasing the heat and light of another earth's climate, dug by dead hands.

Those making that future, buried in the earth to dig in the dark, are paid by the number of cars they load, but only the large contractors and scab miners get the good veins and enough cars. The good practical miner who works carefully and pays his dues gets the bony veins laced with slate, which means working twice as hard for half the money. They order you to load five cars but won't even give you four. Why work blind in thick smoke waiting for cars that never come? Instead get a ride out of the mine in a car hoisted up the shaft. Emerge dizzy from the methane. Blink coal dust from your eyes and then make your way through the colliery yard, past the enormous breaker where sad boys and old men pick slate from the coal under the watchful eye of stick-wielding breaker bosses. Pass the platform men who send the coal out by rail, near the rollercoaster-like track where the dump men and the top men send the coal up to the breaker and the waste material out to the culm pile. Move through the wasteland where firemen in small buildings stoke steam engines that power enormous hoisting gears that turn even larger wheels that haul coal-laden cars up shafts by thick rope; all of it done in the shade of the culm banks, the enormous mountains of waste rock that surround every mine. Walk past the shop where the carloaders attend to the machinery before finally passing through the fortified stockade gate. Follow the trail that leads back to the mine patch. See versions of your future self walking the path with you. The miners with the reddened eyes of those who work buried in the earth, whose faces and hands are pockmarked by the razorlike slivers of coal that seem fired from the earth, like shots from a cop's Winchester rifle. Hear their gasping, asthmatic breathing from a working life spent in powder smoke and coal dust. Watch the slow-motion movement of bodies made arthritic from years spent underground, the result of being frozen then overheated then frozen again, day after day, year after year. Wince with them as they grimace from the lumbago provoked by years shoveling coal half-stooped, from decades spent in the dark on knees pickaxing an unyielding coal face. Give a wide berth to the old-timers who walk funny, who stop short to cough and catch their breath, who when they die some doctor cuts them open and digs deep into them, pulling parts out of them, turning their deaths into a show-and-tell. Look, a lung. See how black it is. Watch it sink in water, like a rock.

As you walk along the path to the mine patch, see the Polish and Lithuanian women and young girls wandering through hazel and huckleberry. Their heads are down, and their hands form lap pouches out of their simple pleated dresses, in which they hold their harvest of nuts and berries. You walk among Pennsylvania's diaspora of landless peasants from Galicia, beet farmers from Bohemia, half and quarter peasants from the Carpathian highlands, Croatian farm laborers who fled to Pennsylvania from vineyards destroyed by pests, refugees from villages along the Dalmatian coast and everywhere along the way north to the Baltic Sea. People who once worked long, scattered ribbons of land *so narrow they had to walk on their neighbor's land to lead the plough horse on their own*. People forced from homelands by land agents brought by the railroads, or scattered by the new taxes that forced them to divide croplands until nothing was left.

They were recruited here by the coal operators to depress the wages and divide the miners. *We want mainly good Italians, Polanders and Hungarians. We do not want any colored help, or Irish, under any circumstances*, say the bosses. They had their mine foremen pay immigrant breaker boys a dollar to write letters home about guaranteed wages and steady work. *We would like to get green labor mostly*, explain the coal presidents, to serve as replacements for all the *undesirable men*, for all the Irish and Welsh miners blacklisted for demanding higher wages, for all those sent away for joining the union. The posters and broadsides of the steamship companies hung in town squares and peasant cottages all over eastern and central Europe. Images of huge ships docking in American ports. Cheap passage, good jobs, free houses. Make money in America. Stay for good or return and buy your land back. Steamship agents and ticket peddlers set up podiums in market towns and offered cut rates for quick passage. But how will I pay? Sell your pigs. I have no pigs. Lease your land to your neighbor. I have no land. Borrow money from your family. They are all gone. Go to the bank and get a loan. And the banks loaned them money because peasants pay their debts. Neighbors pressed photos in their hands when they left. Take this picture of a son or some trusted man. Find him in America. *See if there is still justice in the world.*

They traveled from Trieste or Naples on the Austro-American line, from Fiume on the Cunard line, from Bremen and ports along the Baltic coast, steaming on the wage slave ships of capital. They spent their days on deck smoking and looking at the sky, their nights in crowded steerage-level bunks ignoring fear and fighting nausea. Buy cheap clothes before you leave, they were told. Don't stand out. Some few chose Galveston instead of New York where the immigration agents were said to be easier. Those who came for good went west to Manitoba or the Dakotas and claimed fertile land in the Indian Territories.

Those who arrived in New York found the docks full of agents hiring laborers for the Chicago stockyards, for the New York cigar makers and sugar refineries, for the textile factories in Massachusetts and Connecticut, for the wire and nail factories of Philadelphia. They were offered a dollar and seventy-five cents a day in the Pittsburgh steel mills. Promises of good housing too. Two dollars a day in Cincinnati or Chicago packinghouses, no strikebreaking required, lied the agents. Day after day, week after week, year after year. How much labor does this country need? From steamship to freight train, they were shipped west in a boxcar, like the cattle they would be paid to slaughter. Those who went to the coalfields got their fare paid to Hazleton, where they were told miners got two dollars a day in wages.

Only the lucky ones walked out onto a coalfield train platform and found the man from the photo waiting for them. The rest arrived cold and alone. They slept on the platform next to a small fire they kindled to stay warm. In the morning, they made their way into Hazleton or Shenandoah or Duryea, where they found a Polish or Lithuanian saloonkeeper who let them stay in a bunkroom while they looked for a boardinghouse. They ate boiled pork and drank black coffee while waiting for a Welsh or English contractor to hire them. I'll pay you eighty cents a day, he'd say when he came around, and two days later they found themselves five hundred feet below the earth in a cloud of methane shoveling coal into a buggy by the light of an oil lamp attached to their cap.

No matter where they came from, the newspapers called them Slavs or Huns or Polanders, complained of their uncivilized influence, editorialized for their deportation. The politicians passed laws to limit their options, which had the effect of making their labor cheaper for the coal companies. Children threw stones at them on the street. Constables from the Humane Association came to their homes with questions and left with their children. Deputy sheriffs arrested them and pocketed the fines. These cops, *it ain't law they think about, it's money.* If they came as a family, or a miner started one after he arrived, life was lived in a shanty in one of the mining patches south of Hazleton or west of Shenandoah, or up in Nanticoke in the Wyoming Valley. Fifteen cents a day for a few rooms in a ghetto carved from a ruined forest wedged between a breaker and a burning culm pile. Squalid, hostile places full of nothing built to last. The air smelled like sulfur. The land was blackened and suffocated by culm. The water was thick and black from coal dust. Their wages were swallowed by deductions.

It didn't take them long before they started building their own churches, running their own small shops in the mine patches, commiserating in their own saloons. Saloons on every block because each served as a kind of community center where you could find a friendly face, get a job, where a daughter could mail letters home, where a widow could get a loan, where a striker could book passage back to Europe. They worked hard for pennies a day, hoarding their money. In 1900 they sent nearly four million dollars back to Italy, Polish Russia, and Austria-Hungary. Even during a strike, with no wages, the Hazleton miners sent fifty thousand dollars a month to Europe.

Some in the union despised them, condemned them as untrustworthy, unreliable, blamed them for taking their jobs and lowering their pay. The union leaders said the Slavish *are more lawless than the other miners.* They are *more difficult to control than the English-speaking people.* The United Mine Workers lobbied to have them barred from the country or at least barred from mining. Their presence depressed wages, they said, made organizing difficult and solidarity near impossible. Some believed the mine owners when they said similar things. Like when their foremen called them un-American, dangerous, murderous, hard to handle. *We cannot talk with these people.* Every time the union launched a strike, it ended with more blacklists.

And every blacklisted miner was replaced with an immigrant miner. The companies hired private detectives and labor agents in Philadelphia and New York to scour the docks for *desirable emigrants* who could be *induced to go into the mines.* Seek out the ones who speak no English. The kind of men less likely *to be strikers and cast-off labor from other mines.* Only when it became clear that they couldn't be stopped from coming, did anyone try to organize them.

But they refused to be organized because to the Slavic miners, everyone else seemed like a boss. What did they have in common with the Irish and Welsh miners who owned their own homes and never worried about eviction? What did they have in common with the English and German contractors who cheated them on their wages? We might earn $2.83, they would explain if asked, but these contract miners try to pay us $2.38 instead. And what happens if we join? What then? They'd seen how the union worked. They'd seen the Irish and Welsh miners put down their tools in one region and then work as a scab in another. The Poles and Lithuanians and Hungarians relied instead on their own solidarity, born from the mutual aid societies they built. They parented their own orphans, pooled their money and paid their own death benefits, used *their heavy fists* to fight for their withheld wages. The coal companies and coal-carrying railroads sharpened these divisions and from them were built the great American fortunes of J. P. Morgan, Andrew Mellon, and Andrew Carnegie, who controlled an industry that fueled every other industry, giving rise to a gilded age of great wealth built on the backs of the anthracite miners.

In the 1890s, when the United Mine Workers were smaller than a few hundred dues-paying members, the Slavic miners launched their own work stoppages and waged their own wildcat strikes. Polish and Italian women organized huge marches and parades in the streets. When the coal companies started blacklisting the immigrant miners and replacing them with scabs, the strikers killed the scabs' cows in retaliation. Their boys stoned the scabs' houses. Their girls shunned the scabs' daughters. The women uprooted the scabs' gardens. When storekeepers sold goods to the scabs, the strikers firebombed the merchants' barns and boycotted their shops. When the bosses brought in rough men from Philadelphia to work as Coal and Iron cops, the striking migrants hid in the woods, jumped the cops when they came off the trains, tied them up on the platform, and tossed them in creeks or on the next train back. Maybe, some finally realized, we'd fare better if we joined with the Slavs instead of demanding they join with us.

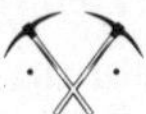

The trail from the mine ends in a mine patch called Jeddo. Find yourself in a front-room saloon in the house of a woman widowed in the last mine disaster. See half-dead Jimmy Gallagher, the Irishman and former Molly Maguire, commiserating at a table with a young miner from eastern Europe. He invites you to sit down, and you take a seat at a small, round table. Jimmy introduces you to Andrew Hannik, his Hungarian neighbor, whose thin face is pockmarked black from coal, same as Gallagher's.

Good afternoon, Andrew, you say. Good afternoon, Jimmy. Get another bobtail check this payday? you ask. I don't even look anymore, says Jimmy. *It is a long time since I know'd in Jeddo how we were paid. Some says we are paid by the ton, and some says we are paid by the car, but how we are paid, I don't know. We get so much for the car anyhow. The car is allowed to be two and three-quarter tons, but I would rather say it is a four-ton car.* They're growing bigger every year, someone says. Gallagher laughs and agrees. *You can put an eleven-foot plank inside the car now, and close the door.* Someone says, at least you're alive, Jimmy, to which Jimmy says loudly, *unless a man is half-killed, he is not hurt.* A few miners at other tables turn toward Jimmy and laugh. One of them says, remind us again, Jimmy. *How many times you get half killed? Twice*, he says, and now the whole saloon is laughing. When was that first time you half-died, Jimmy? you ask. He tells you it was the time with Henry Coll when they mined on the new slope. Yessir, he tells you. We *was the first party that was put down there, to drive an airway, so as to circulate some air through there, so that the men could come in there to work when the place would be ready.* I know that place, says another miner. Air's no good there. Jimmy agrees. That's what me and Andrew been talking about. *Bad air and black damp. I've been carried out several times all but dead.* How often? you ask. *I could not say altogether how often. I know of three times that my own son pulled me out. I knew I was overcome myself, and I could not stand, and he would catch me. My own son worked with me as a laborer. I done the same with him.* Andrew agrees. *Every evening we were not able to get out of the mines it has so much effect on me. I was hardly able—It makes my eyes run water all the time and makes them red.*

Jimmy returns to his story. *I was working four-handed with Henry Coll. We had to go away down through what we called a trial slope—but this day the main slope was open, and the rails was laid on it. There was what they called a feed car. That was not a man car, but a feed car, and the meaning of a feed car is the car that they put the coal on.* He explains that the sides of a feed car hinge open so the coal can be dumped into the chutes at the top of the breaker, which makes it dangerous for a miner to ride down in. But it was the only way down that day, so Jimmy and Henry loaded themselves into the car and then a *man by the name of Kennedy give three raps that was the signal of men coming down. The engineer lowered us down in the car there as carpenters yet working on the place. A block from the carpenter rolled down the plane, halfway or more than halfway down the slope.* The block wedged itself in the rail ahead of them. It got *jammed between one of the center props and the rail.* To make matters worse, he explains, *the slope was not in operation at the time.* Instead of two ropes attached to the car, which stabilizes it as it descends, the car had only a single rope. As the car careened down the rail, approaching the block, it was kind of *shifting backwards and forwards, because it had no other car on to balance it.* That's a steep slope, I know it, says Andrew. Yessir, says Jimmy. And *the car struck this block and jumped off, and of course the engineer slackened.* The slackening made it worse. *The car turned again and went right down the road, and when I seen her, I jumped off.* But instead of continuing down the slope, the car jerked and swung wildly, pinning Jimmy against the wall of the slope. The large hook on the car where the eyebolt of the lift rope connects to the car crashed squarely against him. *I lay there unconscious for a good while.*

The superintendent of the place was the first man who came by and lifted me, and he was the man that got this block out of the way, so the Company could not deny but it was through the fault of the Company that I got hurted. How badly were you hurt? you ask. *Four of my ribs split off the backbone. The superintendent drove me to the doctor. I would not allow them to call an ambulance for fear of exciting and scaring the family.* Henry Coll got it just as bad. Walks the way he does because of it, he says. *There was a tie roller there, and when the car give a sudden jerk against the block*, the hinged door on the hind end opened. Gallagher takes his feet from the floor and places them on the cross piece that connects the feet of the chair you're sitting on. Henry *had his feet the way I have mine against the chair here. He had them against the door that way, and of course she was coming down the pitch where the weight was right on his feet, and when the door flew open his feet ran out and the door came down on him below his knees and smashed his two legs.* That was the first time I got half killed. *Of course, the other story is more simpler to tell.* Let me guess, you say. A roof fell on you. Yessir, he says. Simple as that. *It kind of made me more stooper than what I was before, more humplier-like.*

At that moment, as if he timed it, Henry Coll limps into the saloon and everyone bursts out laughing. Jimmy, with his two feet, kicks out a chair for Henry. I'm telling the story of that time we got thrown from the car, he says. You ask Henry if that was the worst he'd ever been injured too? Been so many, he says, as he sits down. Hard to say. *I got one that nearly finished me. I haven't a safe bone in my body only my neck and that was hurt. My back was hurt too, I have a leg no better than a wooden leg, my ribs are broke, I have only one eye, and my skull is fractured.* How'd you lose the eye? you ask. *A piece of coal hit me in the eye, and it got sore and I had to go to the hospital in Philadelphia and have it taken it out or I would lose the other one.* So that's a glass eye? someone asks. Yes sir, a glass eye, he says. But ain't a good one as I can't see much with it. You scan the room, looking at the miners' laughing faces and realize that the saloon has filled up since you've arrived. It's full of people you've never seen before, which always happens before a strike. The sudden appearance of strange men who want to buy you a beer and ask you questions. Snitches and undercover Pinkertons smoking cigars and drinking beer with talkative miners.

Jimmy gives a soliloquy about how coal cannot be found in the earth. It's not a thing made in the earth, but a thing conjured by the demands and barking orders of the bosses, so many bosses, those rotten souls of capital. Superintendents and assistant superintendents and foremen on the surface and foremen underground and assistant foremen on the surface and assistant foremen underground and driver bosses, and fire bosses, and pump bosses, and door bosses, and docking bosses, and breaker bosses. Bosses managing miners who look made of the earth, as if the earth coughed them up and the bosses and their cops forced them back into the earth. Bosses who call the miners unreliable, sullen, insubordinate, and lazy, as if someone else mines all that coal. Bosses who complain that the miners are married to women who are also lazy and with whom they have children just to have someone to *support the parents in idleness.* The bosses say this on repeat. Tell stories about an entire stratum of people toiling deep in the earth whom they dismiss as ignorant and unskilled, dangerous and undesirable. They say it to the press, and it gets printed in the papers, gets talked about by shareholders, and joins the long list of their reasons they always want more cops.

You're back out in the street again, standing next to Jimmy and Andrew, watching a mine inspector cross the rutted, dirt road. Look, the Angel of Death. Like a ghost, says Gallagher, *I never seen him until when a man got his leg or arm broke or crushed up. When the man was killed, he was always there.* When a miner is killed in the mine, the bosses call the mine inspector. Usually he arrives, looks around, and then explains to everyone that the miner died because he was careless. Gallagher has questions for him.

Mr. Roderick, ain't it? Remember me?

Sorry, friend. Can't say I do.

I'm the fella from the mine that day the Polish miner Monovie *went in and struck a hole in the bench, and we had not time to get fifty yards away when Monovie was killed. The rubbish all fell down on him.* What was it you said that day? What pronouncement was it you made?

I said, I pronounce that man committed suicide.

Why did you do that? Why did you pronounce that?

On account *of the man was not qualified to work and therefore he killed himself.*

Well, sir, *I am no scholar,* but that don't seem right. *What are the causes that produce most of the accidents?*

Falls of rock. A great many of them are due to carelessness and misjudgment. Most of the accidents *must be attributed to the imprudence or whatever it may be termed, of the victims themselves.*

The imprudence, or whatever, of skilled men?

Familiarity breeds contempt, he says, waving off the question.

You mean to say that men who work a dangerous place, or in a dangerous business, become careless?

Careless, some of them do.

It's your claim *that the constant association with dangerous business has a tendency to make men forget this?*

Yes, I have published that in my report.

Tell us, *what was your business before you became a mine inspector?*

Mine foreman.

Gallagher turns and walks away. What's the use of talking? They spend a few days a year in a mine and think they know better than a good practical miner. As you walk you compare the skills of the miners to those of the bosses. A miner, buried in the earth, learns to survive barn-to-barn by listening to every subtle change in the earth as it heaves under its own weight, as its breath escapes from rock, as its water moves through it. Every vein throws off this or that much black damp, this or that much white damp. Every shot the miner fires provokes another unpredictable chemical transformation of air and water and earth. Every shot ripples through rock, like a wave, and then returns transformed as something different, something unexpected. The good practical miner respects the earth and fears the boss, because it's the bosses who kill the miner, not the earth. Listen to a boss instead of the earth and you'll find yourself driving a tunnel straight up into the bottom of the Susquehanna River.

This is not to say the bosses have no skills, Gallagher says with a smirk. Let us count the ways. Hannik tells you to keep count since you're the one with all the fingers. Left thumb: the many skills and accomplishments of the bosses include the managing of miners to their death. Left forefinger: the skill of having the idea of exhuming a buried apocalypse of a different world and releasing it into the present. Left middle finger: the skill of defining productivity as the number of men killed per tons of coal produced. Left ring finger: the skill of being the innovators of the practice of leaving the dragged-out corpses of poisoned or drowned miners on their own rented shanty floors to be found by newly made widows. Left pinky: the skill of being savvy buyers of squibs and fuses made by little girls in factories that sometimes blow up.

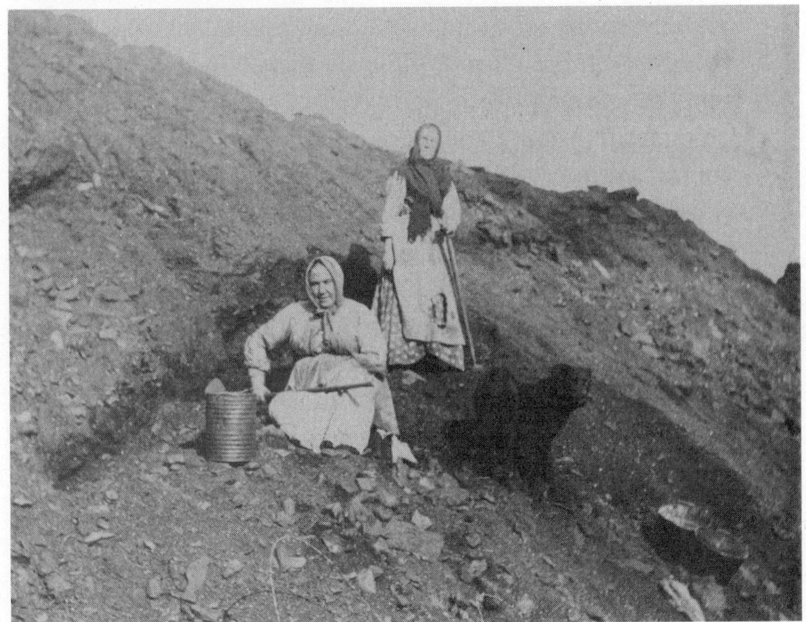

Women collecting coal from a culm bank near Hazleton during the 1902 strike.
Courtesy: Library of Congress.

As you walk, you see a gash in the earth where an abandoned mine has collapsed in on itself, revealing half-buried pillars of coal. An old man carrying a bucket full of coal climbs a ladder out of it. A half mile further on, you see a little girl standing half-buried in a trench dug into a culm pile firing fist-sized rocks to three boys who are catching them on the fly and loading them into a wooden cart. You smile and swivel your head, scanning for the Coal and Iron Police. You're walking to the union hall and talk turns to the strike of 1900, the year the union won a 10 percent wage increase in the six-week strike that turned John Mitchell, the young president of the even-younger United Mine Workers of America, into a household name. What a thing, Gallagher says, that a miner gets called by the president of the United States, gets himself cheered at train depots, trailed by reporters. Imagine a man like Mitchell, who actually knows something about coal mining, living a life like that. Born in Braidwood, Illinois, Mitchell followed his father into the mines at twelve years old and spent his boyhood underground, opening and closing the huge wooden doors that control a mine's ventilation. At sixteen years old, he joined the Knights of Labor, his first introduction to union organizing. He spent the early 1890s laying in water scraping coal from inside a doghole bench, never making more than $750 a year. Must have thought something of himself though, because he spent his nights studying law by the light of an oil lamp, and by the time he was twenty-six, he was working full-time as a labor organizer. By thirty years old, in 1899, he was the president of the United Mine Workers of America. He is the hero of 1900 but if someone tells you the strike was a great victory for the miners, don't believe them. After the strike, the coal operators evicted whole families from company homes, blacklisted coal miners for demanding higher wages, for hollering Scab! at the men who took their jobs, and for stoning the Coal and Iron Police. The miners who kept their jobs found docking bosses even more aggressive and prices for their supplies in the company stores even higher—sky-high rates for black powder and steeper prices for oil.

At least it wasn't 1900 anymore; or 1901 either, which was the year 150,000 hard-rock miners at the hundreds of collieries throughout eastern Pennsylvania dug more hard coal from the earth—sixty million tons—than in any previous year, a number published in every newspaper and mining report and praised in every church sermon, as if that was the number that mattered most. Sixty million tons is a bosses' number, as any good practical miner knows. A number that counts only what the bosses count. A good practical miner counts it differently: 1901 was the year 150,000 miners, with only hand tools and mules and on wages that averaged a dollar a day, hauled out of the earth enough coal, slate, and dirt to cover the entire region in a coalfield-sized culm mountain nearly two hundred feet tall. It was the year the miners pumped enough water from the mines to drown the entire anthracite coalfields in a flood two miles deep. It was the year their sons, sitting all day in clouds of dust in enormous breakers patrolled by angry breaker bosses, sorted actual mountains of earth into coal. It was the year their daughters, little girls thin as reeds, worked third shifts in lace mills and squib factories so their families could afford food. It was the year widows, mine wives, and old women ran boarding houses, cooked and cleaned, gathered berries and nuts, raised chickens, milked cows, and made a stockpile of clothes in case husbands or sons died in the mine. It was the year more miners than ever before joined the United Mine Workers of America, a union cobbled together not more than a decade earlier from all the snitch-destroyed and private-detective-infiltrated unions that preceded it.

Today is May 11, 1902, the day hundreds of local chapters of the United Mine Workers of America will decide whether to refight the strike of 1900. It's said Mitchell opposes another strike, though he's not the only miner who fears it. Mitchell, as everyone knows, fears all strikes. Capital and labor, as he liked to say, are just two intertwined sides *whose interests are so inseparably allied.* But Mitchell couldn't convince the coal companies of this (or most of the miners either). The coal presidents refused to believe that UMW was the conservative, business-minded union he promised it was, despite all the editorials he wrote exclaiming it, all the articles he penned for magazines extolling it, and all the interviews he gave to reporters promising it. He gave speeches in fancy boardrooms explaining how UMW signed binding contracts with coal companies in Illinois, which proved UMW was a partner with capital, not its antagonist. He openly touted the benefits to the coal companies of *our methods of disciplining our members*, and *the reasonableness and conservativeness of our officers.* He reminded the bosses that UMW honored contracts, called no sympathy strikes, ordered miners back to the mines if they disobeyed their foremen. We respect the property rights of the coal companies, he made sure to always say. Made a big thing about how he'd tied the prospects of the UMW to the National Civic Federation, a reformist group of Republican politicians and labor leaders who advocated for industrial stability through conservative, business unionism and who believed that agreements between capitalists and workers were the only way to stop the constant strikes and bloody labor disputes.

When none of it worked, and the miners grew restless, Mitchell brought union leaders, national organizers, and local union delegates to Shamokin, downriver from Wilkes-Barre, in March of 1902, to determine the union's demands. They wanted union recognition (no more handshake agreements), shorter hours and higher wages, a reduction in contracting (no miner should hire more than three laborers), the abolition of the miners' ton, and a multiyear contract. We'll embarrass the coal companies with our willingness to compromise, Mitchell promised. We'll be reasonable and try all conservative measures. For once, he reminded everyone who would listen, we have public opinion on our side and the National Civic Federation in our corner. But the presidents of the coal companies and the coal-carrying railroads saw no upside to acknowledging the authority of the union. *I am anxious to have one thing clearly understood*, said George Baer, the influential president of the Pennsylvania and Reading Railroad, the largest coal-carrying railroad, *we will not deal with that organization.* Some coal-company presidents taunted the miners' union. We hope they go on strike. *We'll save money on the wages of the miners and on the increased prices of the product. While we do not want a fight, we will give the men all the fight they want if they decide that there is to be one.*

When no coal company would even meet with Mitchell, the union's executive committee met in Scranton in early May 1902 and voted sixteen to twelve to call a temporary strike. Fifteen hundred people waited in the street outside Scranton's Carpenter's Hall for news of the vote. The minute the Scranton miners heard it, they canceled their orders for more powder and oil and then went into the mines and brought out their tools, taking them home, oiling them up, and then burying them behind chicken coops for safekeeping. Mitchell ordered each union local to vote on whether to make the strike permanent and to elect a delegate to represent it at a convention in Hazleton, where miners from every local would meet to decide whether to go on strike.

You follow Gallagher and Hannik into the Jeddo union hall and listen to the miners complain in four languages about docking and the lack of cars. Everyone tells a different version of the same story. Miners, *after entering the mines at seven in the morning, have laid there until two o'clock without receiving a mine car. They laid there up to two o'clock on account of a wreckage in that part of the mine. And if they attempted to go home before that time, they would be suspended that day or probably two or more in addition to that. If they laid there from dinner time until ten minutes to five, and then started to go home, and they met the mine driver three quarters of a mile further, with a trip of cars going to their place, if they failed to go back that carried with it a suspension of three days.*

You listen to them talk about the blacklists, of which *there is a standing one in Coxe Brothers Company. A man will be blacklisted for refusing to work on a place of work that they say he must work whether it pays him or not*, says the district president William Dettery. For doing that, *you are blacklisted under that company for six months, and you cannot get any work at any other colliery under that company. I have had my leg and arm broke and I have been hurt across the back. . . . I have worked with two men in my time that were killed, and when I was injured myself there was myself and two laborers injured with me. I have helped to carry hundreds of men from the mines during explosions, helped to rescue them, not only where I live now but in Schuylkill County. . . . I am subject to asthma*. The local treasurer, Paul Dunleavy, says its true at G. B. Markle & Co. too. Markle uses the company houses to get me to work shit jobs, he says. *A man has to take any kind of a place that is given him, if he is not in a position to move*. If he refuses to work a bad breast, he gets evicted and blacklisted. What's the use of working even a good breast? says another man. You'll just get docked for loading light no matter how high you top the cars. Henry Shovlin agrees and says he knows they collect the coal that falls from their cars when hoisted out. It's true, he says. *I was informed by the people that works at the bottom of the slope, such as the man that hauls at the bottom of the slope, that every day at noon they loaded from one car to two cars of coal*. That's our coal, hollers another man. They even make money from us after we die, says Charlie Helferty, the local union president. You all know Kate Burns, right? The widow of the man run over by the lokie engine. It took her and her sons twelve years to pay off what Markle said they owed him. Andrew Chippie too, says another. After his father was killed, he was forced to take the man's place, but never made a dime. A Hungarian miner named Mike Midlick says it ain't like making a wage makes any difference anyway. I got laid off, he says, but *I did not apply any other place because I did not have any money to go anywhere; I went as far as I could go.*

The bosses throw greenhorns into the mine and don't care if they live or die, Dettery says. *In my experience a good practical miner—it will take him at least fifteen years to become efficient in all the different kinds of work that he is called upon to perform. . . . He must know how to make timber, how to stand timber, how to open the chute, how to stand timber in the chute, how to drive the cross chutes, how to put in stumpings and cross cuts, and everything else, standing props and pigeon rests and batteries. . . . A man should know not only how to take care of himself where he comes in contact with gas, but he should also know how to be able to take care of his neighbor at the same time. . . . He should know how to handle all different explosives. . . . I have worked as a miner for seventeen years and I, like many of my fellow craftsmen, do not know half of it yet.*

A young man says he's worked only two years in the mine and figures he'll be an old man before he knows what he's doing. *And you won't have it all learned then either,* says a man named Strannix. A young-looking man says he was fired for kicking a mule that bit him, but the fire boss who never checks for gas still has a job. A stooped-over old-timer who picks slate all day so as to afford a bed at a boarding house says he made better wages during the war. A man in the back says something about how it don't seem worth getting married, what with the misery. Another disagrees. *I wish I was. I was once, but my partner has gone away; she is dead.* Dettery says he heard the head doctor of the Lauryton poor house in Luzerne County say that *about 70 percent* of everyone in the asylum *has chronic rheumatism.* Something like *40 percent are cripples.* The doctor said *they have compound fractures and bruises and crushes of the legs and are crippled on account of that. There are one-armed men and one-legged men, men who have had amputations.* Back injuries, head injuries, melancholy. *There are two there that have been there for two years, lying on what they call a water bed, as the result of mine accidents, lying there with no power at all, just lying there waiting for death.*

The miners elect Charlie Helferty as their delegate at the Hazleton convention, where he will join with hundreds of other delegates at the Grand Opera House debating the strike question on their behalf. And then, with the image in everyone's head of two miners lying in beds made of water waiting for their deaths, the Jeddo miners vote unanimously to lay down their tools and go out on strike.

CHAPTER TWO

A MINERS' TIMELINE

1690 The First Settlers Arrive in the Coalfields and Describe It This Way

William Penn, benevolent utopian sovereign of the settlement, looks north from Philadelphia, into the rugged and forested barrier ranges and beyond and speaks of *communication by water* between the Schuylkill and Susquehanna Rivers.

1737 The First Property Claim to the Coalfields, Backdated

The year of the miraculous finding of the forgotten Treaty of 1686 that white settlers claim converted a million acres of Lenni Lenape homelands to the private property of the heirs of William Penn. The phrase Walking Purchase refers to the way Penn's son, Thomas, established the property's boundary. It is said that upon finding the so-called deed, which described the property's length as a day's walk east from the confluence of the Delaware and Lehigh Rivers, Thomas Penn, who claimed Pennsylvania as his inheritance, hired men to blaze a straight trail through the woods, on which he sent his three fastest runners, with a prize to the one who covered the most ground.

American law traces all claims of private property on this land to this day and to this foot race. Twenty-first-century court challenges to Penn's deed have rejected Native claims of fraud in the acquisition of this land. Fraud, duplicity, and forgery do not invalidate title when land is taken from Native nations, say the courts. This is not surprising since, as the US Supreme Court has declared, *Conquest gives a title which the Courts of the conqueror cannot deny.* For generations to come in the coalfields, foot racing, along with other blood sports such as cockfighting, dog fighting, and pigeon shooting, remain a popular pastime.

1790 The Story of the Hunter Who Discovered Anthracite

Necho Allen, lonely hunter and trapper, kindled a fire at a rocky spot near the Little Schuylkill River. It is said his campsite can be found below Broad Mountain, north of present-day Pottsville, in the rugged and forested terrain of Pennsylvania's Valley and Ridge region, a physiographic area defined by its parallel and plunging synclines and anticlines, its long, folding ridges laced with thick seams of metamorphosed sedimentary rock—anthracite!—of the Carboniferous period, detritus of the tectonic cataclysms, impossible pressure, and intolerable heat of an earth that tore itself apart and then reassembled itself over the course of more than two hundred million years. Broad Mountain begins miles east of where Allen is said to have camped, just west of the Walking Purchase confluence, near the looted toolstone quarries of its first peoples, where the sweep of the Lehigh River carves a deep gorge of riverwashed soils. This future coalfield of forested and folding ridges begins low on the land and then races up and away from the gorge on a west-southwest path, bringing red and white oak with it, on its way to a wild and desolate plateau of stony and shallow soils. It was here, near this high ground, near the present-day settlement of Hazleton, where Allen awoke to find that his fire had set an outcropped rock ablaze. The first to set the earth on fire.

1791 The Last Great Coalfield Defeat of the American Army

The Battle of a Thousand Slain, known also as St. Clair's Defeat or the Battle of the Wabash River, is the story of another group of coalfield hunters. In October 1791, with orders from President George Washington to enter the coalfields and exterminate the Miami nation by blood and fire, Major General Arthur St. Clair marched north from near present-day Cincinnati with two thousand soldiers and a traveling brothel, leaving a line of supply posts and military forts in his wake. As they marched, the crises of conscience and cowardly desertions that plague all settler armies winnowed his forces. Frequent ambushes by Native reconnaissance forces thinned them further. He established a camp on the evening of November 3 on the high ground above the headwaters of the Wabash River. A thousand Native fighters waited in ambush below them. As snow fell under darkening skies, the great Miami leader Mishikinaakwa moved his warriors from their hidden positions into a crescent-shaped fighting line across the Wabash from St. Clair's camp. Ojibwe, Pottawatomie, and Ottawa fighters, with the Ottawa Chief Egushaway in the lead, moved into positions to the west. Shawnee and Lenape warriors, with the Lenape leader Buckongahelas among them, took up fighting positions to their flank. To the northeast, a force of Seneca, Cherokee, and Wyndot lay in wait. It is said Egushaway, Buckongahelas, and the Shawnee war chief Waweyapiersenwaw deferred to Mishikinaakwa, who led the combined forces in battle. When the shooting began at sunrise, under clear skies, some soldiers turned, ran, found themselves surrounded, and were killed. Gunners swiveled their field artillery into place but could only fire weakly into trees. Their officers fell to Native snipers. The gunners were killed as they spiked their guns. Militiamen hid in tents and pretended to be women, pleading for their lives. None received mercy. A thousand US soldiers died in the battle. St. Clair, asleep when the shooting started, or so he claimed, survived. The battle marked the worst military defeat of the armies of the United States in all the battles in all the wars it waged against all Native nations. With two dozen others, St. Clair lived to tell tales of his innocence and of Native savagery, fuel for future campaigns of revenge.

1791 The First Record of Commercial Anthracite Mining

With the American Army in the coalfields, the Lehigh Coal Company declared itself, opened a mine, built a rough road to the river, and launched rafts and arks of coal through rapids and over falls, nearly all of which stoved on rocks and broke apart, returning the coal to the earth.

1813 The Beginning of the Era of Inland Commerce

The year armed woodhicks along the Susquehanna, the Lehigh, and the Schuylkill rivers converted forests of white pine trees into tall, straight spars, which they sold to ark builders, who mortised them together into ark hulls, which they held fast by oak or ash pins. On these hulls the ark builders pegged pine planks together to make decks whose seams they waterproofed with cotton or flax mixed with pitch or tar. On these rough decks, they built shanties for cargoes of wheat, pigs, whiskey, coal, and as shelter for oarsmen. These arks were useless until the floods of the spring freshet opened a small window for the two-handed crews to scramble into swift water.

The sight of the arks—hundreds a day during the spring floods—brought settlers to the banks to watch the lumbering vessels run rapids past grist mills and sawmills. They took up positions along the most treacherous sections of the river and waited for the arks to break apart against the rocks, whereupon they made off with their cargoes. If the pilots made it to market, they sold the cargo, disassembled the arks, parted out the lumber, kept the nails, and walked back to do it again.

All agreed this was no way to make an industry. Nothing could be taken to market until the brief spring freshet turned impassable rivers into barely navigable ones. To develop inland commerce and grow industrial capacity, river navigation would have to be made reliable and year-round. To this end, navigation companies announced themselves and secured monopoly charters from the state, which they used to entice investors. With firms capitalized, engineers and surveyors appeared along the Lehigh and its tributaries, the Susquehanna and its branches, and the Schuylkill and Little Schuylkill Rivers. They hiked along rocky riverbanks thick with ash and alder trees carrying long rods with them, which they used to take measure of the river. Their reports identified which boulders to be hauled away, which overhangs to be removed, and where water levels needed to be raised. They noted locations for the placement of chutes, calculated the orientation of angled dams, and noted the proper location of slackwater ponds. They built canals where the rivers resisted improvement, converting water and land into a network of tollways under their control.

Instead of relying on the crude roads that connected their mines to rivers or canals, which were often impassable in winter and impractical as the tonnage grew, they built rollercoaster-like funiculars that worked through the pairing of counterbalanced cars. As a loaded car of coal descended from mine to river, it drew up an empty car on a parallel track. With transportation secured, they printed handbills in English and German and went door to door, business by business, publicizing their innovations in transportation and stove design. In the southern fields, the operators shipped coal on the Schuylkill Canal from Pottsville to Philadelphia. In the northern Wyoming Valley, the Delaware and Hudson Canal Company floated rafts and arks along a route to Rondout in New York and then on to the Hudson River. The Pennsylvania Canal ran from Nanticoke to Sunbury and then to Port Deposit over the Chesapeake and Tidewater Canal. The Lehigh Canal traveled riverside from Mauch Chunk to Easton and then on to Philadelphia through the Delaware Division Canal, or to Perth Amboy in New Jersey via the Morris Canal.

By 1825, the rivers and canals brought nearly 35,000 tons of anthracite to tidewater, a number that for the first time exceeded imported coal. By 1832, more than 1,500 watercraft carried 158,000 tons of stone coal to market. By 1836, more than 3,000 rafts brought 345,000 tons to market. By 1840, the Schuylkill Navigation Canal dominated the anthracite trade, dictating shipping rates throughout the coalfields. But it would not last. In 1842, the Philadelphia and Reading Railroad built track on routes that paralleled the canals. At first, competition among the canal and railway companies developed in almost complementary fashion, but soon the railroads expanded and built trunk and feeder lines. Their spurs ran directly to the breakers. The Schuylkill Canal invested in new docks and landings and widened and deepened its canal, which doubled its traffic, allowing it to lower its shipping costs, but the cost of these improvements drowned it in debt. By the 1850s the Pennsylvania and Reading dominated shipping along the Schuylkill. The Lehigh Valley Railroad took freight from the Lehigh Canal. The Delaware, Lackawanna & Western Railroad hijacked Wyoming Valley shipping. Anthracite mining was now a wholly owned subsidiary of the railroads. Only a handful of independent operators remained. The rest were eventually absorbed into J. P. Morgan's coal trust.

1828 The First Report of the Miners' Wages

A dollar a day. Laborers get eighty cents.

1845 The First Report of a Fatal Rockfall

The day—June 5, 1845—when sixty tons of earth in the Hollenback Coal Mine collapsed onto Joseph Walker, John Carey, and fifteen-year-old John O'Neal, killing them instantly. The miners were blamed for their deaths.

1845 The First Report of an Explosion That Didn't Kill a Miner

The August day in 1845 when the miners of the Delaware Coal Company in Schuylkill County refused to enter the gaseous, three-hundred-foot-deep West Mine. Upon their refusal the mine's overseers descended into the earth to prove the miners wrong, whereupon the flames of their oil lamps ignited the firedamp, triggering an explosion that destroyed the underground workings and nearly killed them all.

1847 The First Report of a Fatal Explosion

The day—April 13, 1847—that the Hollenback Coal Mine exploded and killed the miner John Zeigler. The miner was blamed for his death.

1848 The First Benevolent Society Organized in the Collective Interests of the Miners

The Bates Union, named after its founder, the English chartist John Bates, organized five thousand mine workers in Schuylkill County. Its first campaign focused on the miners' complaints of excessive docking and coal-car topping. Bates declared a strike in 1849, the first organized work stoppage by coal miners in the United States, which collapsed after three weeks, whereupon he absconded with the miners' dues and was never seen again.

1855 The Year Anthracite Replaced Charcoal as an Industrial Fuel

The turning point came during the British Royal Navy blockade of all maritime traffic along the Eastern Seaboard during the War of 1812, when American merchants and industrialists, starved of imports, turned their attention inland, to the vast coalfields of eastern Virginia and eastern Pennsylvania. By the time the first shots were fired in the Civil War, their network of newly built canals and railroads, their improvements in stoves, and the arrival of steam engines, first built in 1813, transformed anthracite into a crucial domestic and industrial fuel. It would be during the Civil War, however, that anthracite became something more than an industrial fuel. *The United States should at once possess itself of the entire anthracite field of Pennsylvania*, wrote a former admiral of the Union Navy, *and retain it for purposes of national defence.* This was not a fuel, it was a weapon, a guarantee of security, unmatched anywhere in the world. No other country possessed such a weapon and in such vast amounts. Anthracite burned without producing the familiar ribbonlike curl of black smoke that usually marked a ship's location, which allowed Union warships to slip undetected into southern ports and creep ghostlike along Confederate shores. Some said anthracite won the war, and those who did declared stone coal a transformative weapon of abolition. What burden can't this fuel free us from? What earthly limit can't it transcend? Its use grew from a few hundred tons in the first years after the War of 1812 to more than a million tons by 1837.

1860 The First Miners' Union to Organize the Entire Coalfields

A tumultuous decade of labor organizing began with the formation of a series of regional societies beginning with the Forestville Improvement Society of 1860. This was followed by the Miners' Benevolent Society of Locust Gap, which predated the Archibald Benevolent Association of 1863, which came the year before the Benevolent Society of Carbon County, all of which culminated in the legendary John Siney's Workingmen's Associations of the Anthracite Fields of Pennsylvania, also known as the Workingmen's Benevolent Association, or WBA, which started small but then grew as it absorbed the smaller, regional societies that preceded it.

Siney improved working conditions and wages for the miners by lobbying for legislation that eroded the authority of the docking bosses. But he was no militant labor leader. His WBA sought a capital-friendly business unionism. Like many of the union leaders who would follow him, he did not see the coal bosses as the miners' antagonists. Instead, he saw the problem of low wages and dangerous working conditions as a market problem, a product of the boom-and-bust nature of the industry. His strategy, common still today, was to organize mine workers into a labor cartel and then rent this cartel to industry in return for higher wages. This, he claimed, would stabilize the price of coal and solve the miners' problems. For it to work, the miners would have to throw themselves out of work when prices dropped.

A second and equally intractable problem that confronted Siney was the difficulty of building an organization of mine workers that accounted for the regional differences that divided them. The complaints of miners in one valley rarely overlapped with the complaints of miners in another. When the Schuylkill miners, who worked the hard, pitching, difficult-to-near-impossible veins of the southern fields, complained of excessive docking and topping and laid down their tools, they were replaced by the northern miners who shared only some of those conditions and held different grievances. These contradictions, which would eventually doom the WBA, were briefly suspended during the Civil War, when wages and prices spiked with the onset of fighting. By 1865, contract miners made $150 to $200 a month, some more. Mine laborers, among the worst paid workers before the war, became among its best paid during it. The war's end brought waves of investment and a flood of returning miners who competed for rapidly declining wages. When Siney declared a strike in 1869, it was the first time that miners from every region walked out as one. Siney, however, proved unprepared for a long struggle and when the Wyoming Valley miners saw their interests ignored in favor of the Schuylkill miners, they agreed to terms that benefited only them, and the strike collapsed.

1863 The First Military Occupation of the Coalfields

When the Irish miners, newly organized by a benevolent society known as the Molly Maguires, demanded higher wages, the coal companies, which controlled conscription into the Union Army, depicted them as un-American, and their pickets and parades as having nothing to do with wages or working conditions. It was a treasonous tactic, they claimed, designed to sabotage the Union's war efforts. Provost Marshal Charlemagne Tower, prolific land speculator and coal-mine owner, depicted the Molly Maguires as a terrorist organization and called in federal troops.

1866 The First Coalfield Police

The year Pennsylvania supplemented its industrial police statute by authorizing the governor of Pennsylvania to commission Coal and Iron Police upon the request of companies engaged in the mining of coal or the making of iron. The statute allowed for police specifically for persons in possession of collieries, furnaces, and rolling mills. The act gave individual Coal and Iron Police officers *all the powers of policemen of the city of Philadelphia in the several counties in which they shall be so authorized to act.* The act reserved for the coal companies the right to select and train officers and form units. It left for the state the obligation to commission these police. During times of strike, thousands of Coal and Iron cops patrolled the collieries, each with the legal authority of any cop anywhere. *Their powers are general, as the Act expressly confers the right to arrest all persons engaged in the commission of any offence against the laws of the commonwealth which may be committed on railroad property. In making arrests for the violation of law not immediately concerning property of the railroad company, these officers act not as agents of the company, but as policemen.*

The Coal and Iron Police statute didn't create a standing police agency, it established a public license to raise private armies of strikebreakers. When miners called a strike, the coal operators hired detective agencies in Philadelphia and Baltimore to hire police from among the riffraff and the cutthroats. They shipped these men into the coalfields, where the companies armed them, paid them more than the miners got, and billeted them in barracks next to company-run brothels. They were known to fire into crowds full of children. They were said to use their blackjacks and revolvers at the slightest provocation. The union despised them, children stoned them. In the years after 1902, Progressive-Era reformers called for the abolition of the

Coal and Iron Police because its violence threatened the legitimacy of the state's police powers. Some also worried that *their violence made men communists.*

1870 The First Coal Cartel Stakes a Claim to the Coalfields

Franklin Gowen, the son of Irish Protestant merchants and failed coal-mine operator, came to prominence in the 1860s as the Pottsville district attorney, a position from which he built a lucrative private practice in the quieting of coalfield titles on behalf of railroad interests, particularly the Philadelphia and Reading Railroad, for whom he brokered secret land purchases in violation of the carrier's corporate charter. The board of directors made him its president in January 1870. As president, he used incentives and strong-arm tactics to bind the railroads and coal operators together into a cartel. He then negotiated a deal with Siney known as the Gowen Compromise, which established a standard wage-basis pegged to the price of coal.

When the price of coal increased, operators agreed to raise the miners' wages. When the price declined, the operators were free to cut wages. Siney agreed to the deal because he viewed the interests of miners and operators as shared. The real enemy of working people, Siney told the miners, wasn't the bosses but the unpredictability of the market. According to this way of thinking, the collective demands for higher wages warped the market and disrupted industrial production, which produced increased price and production volatility.

Siney didn't think this logic through, but Gowen did, and he took it to its horrifying conclusion, which was that the persistent demands for higher wages by organized combinations of workers constituted a willful violation of the law of the market. After all, if the market dictated wages, and those wages were paid to miners whose labor made industrialism possible, it was not surprising the bosses would believe that the market was the source of industrial society itself. Using this logic, it was not a stretch for the bosses to claim that the wage demands of workers did more than just warp the market, it threatened the very fabric of society itself. This is why the bosses refused to recognize combinations of labor. If workers were allowed to organize, they would use that power to dictate wages, and if workers dictated wages, they would control the market. And if they controlled the market, the world would be theirs. The solution, according to Gowen, was to stop their organizers, and the most effective way to do that was to eliminate them, which Gowen spent his entire adult life trying to do.

This strategy began in 1871, when Gowen stage-managed an industry-wide tripling of freight rates, which devoured the profits of the coal companies still independent of Gowen's cartel. The independent operators cut wages, which provoked waves of wildcat strikes, walkouts, and work stoppages, which led to a collapse in coal production.

Gowen, anticipating all this, secretly created a front company called the Laurel Run Improvement Co., which he used to buy up all the companies bankrupted by his freight rates. He then evaded the law that prohibited railroads from owning collieries by creating another front company called the Philadelphia and Reading Coal and Iron Company. He named himself president and purchased all shares of Laurel Run. By 1874, this front company, along with the coal-carrying railroads, controlled the production and shipping of nearly the entire anthracite industry. Siney declared a general strike in the coalfields. Gowen pretended to capitulate to the miners' demands, enticing them back to the mines with a small wage increase and vague promises of future negotiations. When mining resumed, Gowen filled his reserves with coal and then flooded the market. He declared the market saturated in November of 1874, which collapsed the price of coal, triggering the Gowen Compromise.

When the miners refused the wage cuts, he closed the mines and locked them out. His cartel of coal-carrying railroads then announced it would not purchase or ship the coal of the few remaining independent coal companies, which had the intended effect of locking out all remaining miners. He then offered to reopen the mines and resume shipments but only if the miners agreed to a 20 percent wage cut.

This was the start of the months of misery known as the Long Strike of 1875, in which starving miners looked for signs of weakness in the operators' position but found instead a growing army of Pinkertons, Coal and Iron Police, and militia armed to the teeth, hunting them in the coalfields. The striking miners overturned Pennsylvania and Reading trains and set culm banks and colliery stockades on fire. Starving children survived on roots dug from forest floors. Siney and his union, lacking strike funds, eventually agreed to the wage cuts and ordered the miners back to the mines, but Gowen refused to take them. The more the miners suffered, he boasted, the more money he made. By late spring, all was lost. Desperate miners in the Wyoming Valley saw no good end and abandoned the strike. Some took the jobs of starving miners in Schuylkill County. Union leaders blamed the Wyoming miners for the defeat, calling them scabs, blacklegs, and claiming they alone were responsible for this catastrophe. But the defeat was described differently in poems found posted on fence posts and in ballads sung in saloons. It was Siney, his WBA, and all those duped by the Gowen Compromise, who were to blame. Their leaders had sold them out and condemned them to this poverty.

The Ballad of the Blacklegs

What if this union was forsaken forever,
And poor men made slaves as they've been before?
To make matters worse, they must work of small wages;
They ne'er can pay their bills that they owe in the store.
If they had been united and pulled all together,
And kept politics within their own bounds—
But when they were elected, the poor was neglected;
They sold the men's freedom to Franklin B. Gowen.

1870 The First Regional Coalfield Police

The statute that permitted Coal and Iron Police limited police commissions to the county of the employing colliery. By limiting where private police could operate, the statute had the effect of making the police forces of the large operators temporary, defensive, ad hoc, and guard-like in nature. The large cartel of coal-carrying operators raised enormous armies of cops each time there was a strike, disbanding them when the strike ended. The Hazleton-area independent coal companies, however, squeezed by the coal cartel's shipping monopoly, could not afford the expense of raising enormous armies of strikebreaking police strike after strike. As a cost-saving measure, they pooled their funds and created a regional police agency, the North Lehigh Coal and Iron Police Association, which was established as a private, unincorporated, armed police force for the purpose, according to its lawyer, *of rendering voluntary aid to each other in case of trouble.*

During the strike of 1902, the Hazleton-area companies, which operated collieries across three counties (Luzerne, Schuylkill, and Carbon), realized the advantage their regional police agency gave them. When they filed their petitions to the state for police commissions, they filed them as joint petitions, which gave their cops powers greater than those of Philadelphia police. This was because the North Lehigh Coal and Iron Police Association served companies with collieries in three different counties. The North Lehigh cops, therefore, had the authority to patrol beyond each county's boundary, which made it the first regional police agency in the United States. It stored its arsenal of Spencer and Winchester pump-action shotguns, Springfield breech-loading shotguns, Spencer and Winchester rifles, Springfield repeating rifles, and Luger pistols and carbines in the Hazleton warehouse of the Pardee and Co. company store. It ran its intelligence unit and operated a network of snitches and spies out of the Coxe Bros. & Co. clerk's office.

Thereafter, whenever the sheriffs of Luzerne, Schuylkill, or Carbon County sought a posse, they turned to the North Lehigh Coal and Iron Police Association for men and guns. When not riding posse, the North Lehigh cops guarded collieries and protected scabs during strikes. When not on strike duty, it patrolled the primarily Polish, Lithuanian, Hungarian, or Ruthenian mine patches of Drifton, Jeddo, Freeland, McAdoo, and Beaver Meadow, arresting boys for stoning them, men for calling them vile names, girls for gathering culm, women for throwing pots at them, and strikers for sinking bootleg mines.

1873 The First Detective Agency in the Coalfields

The first detective agency in the United States, called the North-West Detective Agency, was founded in 1850 by Allan Pinkerton, the failed barrel maker from England known for a lack of social skills. Pinkerton later changed the name to the Pinkerton Detective Agency, using as its logo an eye encircled by the name of the agency floating above the catchphrase *We Never Sleep,* the image from which the term private eye is derived.

Pinkerton was a Chartist as a young man in England and embraced abolition when he came to the United States. It's said he cried the first time he read Frederick Douglass. Pinkerton, the relentless self-aggrandizer, publicity hound, and pulp fiction writer of lurid stories of the unbelievable exploits of his undercover detectives, is said to have foiled a plot to kill Abraham Lincoln, which he parlayed into prominence. Pinkerton, who spirited escaped slaves to freedom in Canada with John Brown, is said to have served as a foreman on the Underground Railroad. Pinkerton, friend of a friend of Karl Marx, saw no contradiction in his lifelong hatred for combinations of labor. Like many of the white abolitionists and future progressives of his time, he expressed his hatred for slavery through his worship of capital. He celebrated its emancipatory, world-making potential and was awestruck by its unrestrainable drive to replace the slavedriver's lash with the honest day's wage.

Pinkerton saw the wage as the young Frederick Douglass first did. Finally freed from his shackles, in the clothes of a common laborer, Douglass marveled at the sight of two silver half dollars placed in his hands, his first wage. *I was now my own master,* he thought. Though Pinkerton never shook this belief, Douglass came to see the wage's *perpetual whirl of excitement* as nothing but a *slightly less galling and crushing tool of enslavement.* Pinkerton spent his life resisting this insight, devoting it instead to fighting those *black dragons* of terror, as he called the labor organizers, and sending wage workers to jail or to the gallows. This view brought him to the attention of Franklin Gowen, who, seeking to destroy the WBA, hired Pinkerton in October of 1873. Pinkerton sent detectives into the coalfields, where they spent years doing what they called shadow work: tailing working people, loitering in saloons, infiltrating secret meetings. They settled their sights on the Ancient Order of the

Hibernians, known as the Molly Maguires, a secret society of Irish miners that terrorized the coalfield with its militant benevolence for the downtrodden and its burning hatred for the bosses.

1877 The First Mass Execution in the Coalfields

The Day of the Rope, also known as Black Tuesday, was the summer solstice day that ten Molly Maguires, all coal miners, were hanged to death. James Carroll, James Roarity, Hugh McGehan, James Boyle, Thomas Munley, and Thomas Duffy were hanged from a Pottsville prison-yard gallows under a blackening sky. Edward Kelly, Michael Doyle, Alexander Campbell, and John Donahue were hanged from ropes in a Mauch Chunk prison corridor. They were hanged all at once in Pottsville, but since no large gallows could be built inside the Mauch Chunk jail, they were hanged in twos until all were dead. Their families and friends screamed and sobbed as the hangmen led their loved ones to the ropes. Some men declared their innocence from the scaffold, others carried roses to their deaths and said nothing. Newspapers celebrated the day, declaring it good these men were hanged to death, for it was only in the swing of their bodies from rope that *the vindicated majesty of law* could be found. Gowen, who had sent the Pinkertons after them, served as a special state prosecutor in the trials that sent the men to their deaths, convicting them with fantastical stories of murder conspiracies testified to by James McParland, the Pinkerton detective he sent gallivanting around coal country in a flamboyant caricature of an Irish miner.

It is said that in the moments before Alexander Campbell was taken from his cell to the gallows, he grabbed a handful of dirt from the floor and pressed it into the stone wall, making a handprint. I am innocent, he said. Let this mark be *proof of my words.* A hundred years of sheriffs and gallowsmen have scrubbed it off, bleached it away, painted over it, and cut it from stone, but always it reappeared. They knocked the wall down and built a new one, and yet somehow the mark returned, still there today, the haunting mark of a fugitive order.

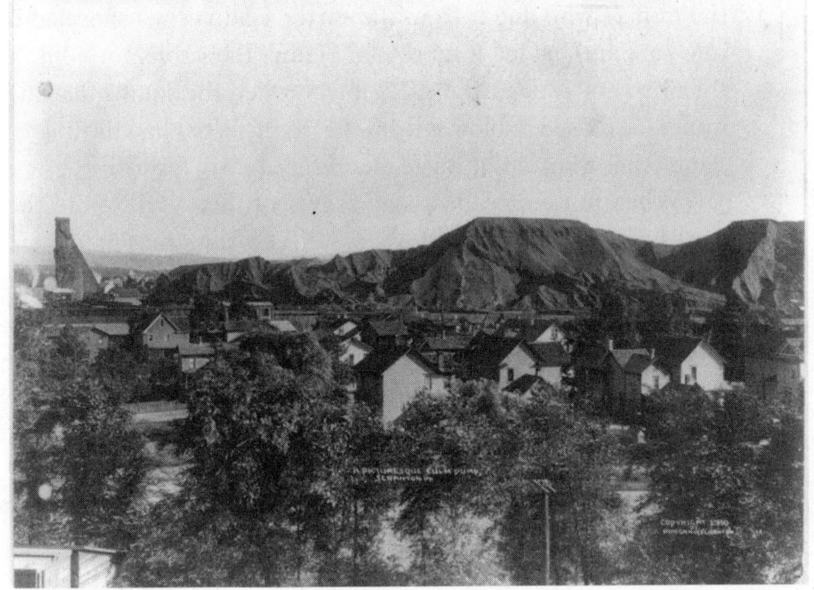

Culm banks looming over Scranton. Courtesy: Library of Congress.

1890 The First Coalfield Washeries Mark the Last Enclosure of the Commons

For generations, the coal operators dumped more than a third of everything the miners dug from the earth into huge, mountains of slate, dirt, and coal called culm banks, those sulfurous mountains of dug-up earth that glowed at night from the light of buried blue flames. They were known to explode spontaneously, like volcanoes, launching dirt, slate, and coal in every direction, giving the land the appearance of a debris field. Rain carried culm into creeks, thickening the water and covering the banks in concentrated sediments of coal dust. Prior to 1886, some operators sold small amounts of cut-rate bony coal to mine workers, but most couldn't afford even this. But no matter, there were always the culm banks, which, like the cave-ins of the abandoned mines, served as a commons, and rightly so. Was it not the miners who dug it from the earth? Hadn't they shoveled it into cars and hauled it up shafts? Hadn't their sons sorted it in the breakers? Hadn't their daughters rolled the squibs that the miners had used to blow it from the earth? What had the bosses done other than call it waste and refuse to pay for it?

When miners needed coal, they sent their children to the banks with shovels and wheelbarrows. Old-timers, injured men, and discarded widows dug into the culm banks, screened it into wagons, and then peddled it on the streets for their survival. But by 1890, when new stove grate designs made the burning of smaller grades of anthracite feasible, the bosses erected no trespassing signs and posted Coal and Iron Police around the culm banks. They laid pipe to dammed creeks and brought water to their newly built washeries, where miners who once worked underground now cleaned and prepared culm for shipment. Some worked on the culm crews that shoveled the culm onto the chutes that carried the rock into the washeries, spending their days in shirtsleeves, even in winter, digging into smoldering culm banks. The chutes deposited the shoveled culm onto the washeries' large, wet concentrating tables where its great agitators separated out the dirt and rock. By 1901, something like 5 percent of all prepared coal sold by dealers began first as culm. By 1911, sales of culmcoal from washeries surpassed the revenue of minecoal. The companies shipped the culmcoal out of the washeries by lokie engine and then discharged the slurry into creeks and rivers, turning every waterway *into a mass of black flowing stuff, . . . a curse to all forms of organic life.*

1890 The First Great Union Arrives in the Coalfield

After the defeat of Siney's Workingmen's Benevolent Association, the Knights of Labor merged with the Miners and Laborers' Amalgamated Association. The new joint union called a strike in 1887 under the banner, *not a drill or pick is used nor a pound of coal mined.* In retaliation, the coal companies evicted miners from company homes, hired scabs to replace the miners, and split union solidarity by offering raises to some miners but not to others. Striking miners suffered a miserable winter on strike and in February, when starving miners began crossing picket lines, union leaders wavered. The strike collapsed completely by mid-March when both unions gave up the fight. The coal companies blacklisted seven hundred miners for their role in the strike, which destroyed the Knights of Labor, leaving only a small subgroup called the National Trade Assembly 135. From this defeat the United Mine Workers of America rose phoenix-like in January 1890, in Columbus, Ohio, when the Assembly agreed to merge with the Coal Miners' and Laborers' National Progressive Union.

1897 The First Massacre of Miners by Coalfield Police

On August 13, 1897, the private secretary of the Lehigh Valley Coal Company threatened to withdraw from the North Lehigh Coal and Iron Police Association. Instead of performing the duty to which the police were assigned, he complained, they acted as a kind of rural, morality police, patrolling the mine patches and paying *entirely too much attention to Hungarian weddings.* The announcement made no mention of the events of the previous day, when Gomer Jones, the superintendent of the Honeybrook Colliery in McAdoo, added two hours of unpaid labor to the teenage muledrivers' workday. When the muledrivers walked off the job, Jones beat a boy with an axe handle, as was his custom. In retaliation, four hundred infuriated miners armed themselves with miners' needles, clubs, knives, and pistols and declared a strike. They marched to surrounding collieries and induced more miners to join the strike. By the end of the week, when the United Mine Workers promised to support their strike, thousands of Polish, Lithuanian, and Hungarian miners joined the union for the first time. When the strike kept spreading, the North Lehigh Coal and Iron Police Association declared its intention to reorganize rather than dissolve. *We need better protection,* they announced. *And we mean to have it.*

By September, tens of thousands of striking immigrant miners organized daily marches to collieries throughout the region. On September 4, the superintendent of Coxe Bros. & Co., L. C. Smith, who also served as the recruiter and purchasing agent for the North Lehigh Coal and Iron Police Association, ordered one hundred Winchester and Spencer rifles and shotguns and had them shipped to the Pardee company store. When they arrived on September 6, Ario Pardee Platt, the manager of the company store and treasurer of the North Lehigh cops, offered them to the sheriff's posse, which the sheriff had formed under pressure from Coxe Bros. & Co. The next day, Sheriff James Martin deputized the entire North Lehigh Coal and Iron Police Association, doubling the size of his posse.

On September 10, striking miners from the Silver Brook colliery marched to West Hazleton and drove off the scabs who had taken their jobs, using their fists to fight off a counterattack by a sheriff's posse detachment. When the scabs ran off and the posse retreated, the marchers headed to Lattimer where they declared their intention to induce the miners there to join the strike. Sheriff Martin raced ahead and blocked the road. *This is a public road*, they said defiantly when they arrived at the blockade, five hundred strong. *We won't leave it until we reach Lattimer.* Martin testified that he read the riot act, but no marcher heard it. He said a man grabbed his gun, though no one saw it. Members of the posse testified later that Martin gave the order to fire, though Martin denied it.

I lay down when the shooting occurred, Fandishaf Maxilon told the coroner, *as I was afraid to run.* From his back, on the road, he watched as the deputies opened fire at Martin's order, shooting men in the back as they ran. Everyone around Maxilon was hit. *I didn't know their names,* he said. *We had no particular leader.* When the firing started, Martin Rosko turned to run but was hit in the arm. Paul Yavock, hiding behind a tree, watched Deputy William Raught shoot a man in the back. A deputy kicked Mike Cheslak to see if he was alive. Survivors dragged wounded men to a nearby schoolhouse or under the shade trees that lined the road. The St. Stanislaus priest moved among the fallen, taking confessions, cleansing souls, and preparing them for the afterlife. When the shooting stopped, searchers looked for survivors by following blood trails up into the mountain, where they found bodies slumped against trees. Eleven died on the road that day and eight more later of wounds. The coroner found that most had been shot in the back. More than three dozen were wounded: Andrew Shabolick survived a rifle shot to the chest. John Kulich took a bullet to the stomach. George Krezo in his leg, hip, and knee. John Damensko and George Vercheck survived rifle shots to both legs.

While the bodies of the injured and dead still filled the road, Martin's deputy sheriff, T. Milner Morris, collected the rifles from the posse and returned them to the Coxe Bros. and Co. Clerk E. A. Oberrender, who returned them to the North Lehigh Association arsenal. Among those who served on the posse were the president, the secretary, the treasurer and the chief of the North Lehigh Coal and Iron Police Association.

1900 The First Reformers Arrive in the Coalfields

The year of the founding of the National Civic Foundation, one of the earliest Progressive-reform institutions in the United States, created to propose political and economic reforms for the making of a new, stable, industrial order. The Republican-Party dominated Federation, which became the UMW's partner and greatest proponent, was part of a broad progressive political movement based on a devotion to capital expressed through demands for quality-of-life reforms designed to create more market-friendly modes of governance.

Progressives supported the combinations of labor of working people, but only if they honored contracts, refused sympathy strikes, disciplined themselves on capital's behalf, and limited grievances to wages and working conditions. Mitchell agreed to it all, in the hope that, in return, organized labor would be allowed to face capital on an equal footing. As he would explain, *it seems to me that the larger and more powerful a labor organization is, the more conservative and safe it becomes.* This idea can be found threaded through all Progressive political thinking. Find it in the Progressive-Era campaign for temperance, which occupied the coalfields with an army of teetotalers. *Industrial harmony,* the temperance advocates explained, *would never flourish until the coal operators have banned liquor from their property.* As the Progressive-Era economist Irving Fisher explained, prohibition *would speed up production probably at least ten percent.* The editor of the influential Pottsville newspaper *The Miner's Journal* claimed that *one-quarter of the work force spent more time in the beer shops than in the mine breasts, costing the coal trade one thousand tons and one thousand dollars a day.* Should this not alarm us? After all *the first requirement for low labor cost production is a healthy contented worker.* Through temperance, we could finally transform the unruly, discontented worker into one suited for the drudgery of factory work.

Progressives also attacked the corruption of the political machines in the cities, or anything that served the interests of those unassimilable immigrant populations that placed a drag on productivity. Let's not be confused, they sermonized, *a large number of the mine workers are not citizens of the country nor do they intend ever to become such. This class does not appreciate or understand our institutions. Brought up under the influence of the bayonet they understand only its restraint. Ignorant, they do not recognize the self-restraint which our free American life makes necessary to the happiness and well-being of our people.* But if we forsake them, the union responded, the communists and anarchists will organize them against us.

A pro-union newspaper once described *the hillsides of Pennsylvania as the most fertile breeding grounds of anarchy and bolshevism.* While there were *no anarchists in the trades union movement,* Mitchell claimed, that will change without the bulwark of conservative unionism. After all, the socialists are holding *immense meetings in every mining town.* We will organize the immigrants already here, he made clear. But enough is enough. *It is my opinion,* Mitchell testified, *that a law should be enacted prohibiting immigration of foreigners at the present time, for the reason that they are not only injuring American working men, but . . . are injured themselves by finding the conditions of employment not as represented to them by the steamship companies who have advertised the favorable and desirable conditions of employment here.*

1902 The Beginning of the Never-Ending Coalfield Strike

After its founding in 1890, the United Mine Workers built local chapters throughout the Wyoming Valley but found only limited success in southern and middle fields dominated by Eastern European miners. In early 1900, union leaders from the Wyoming Valley, where nearly 60 percent of miners had joined the UMW, petitioned Mitchell and the UMW for permission to call a strike. Mitchell refused, pointing to the lack of support among miners from the southern and middle fields. The entire Wyoming Valley is engulfed in wildcat strikes, argued T. D. Nichols, the union leader from the north. Support for a region-wide strike is large and growing. If we don't strike now, he told Mitchell, we'll lose the support of the miners. Mitchell reluctantly agreed but only after the end of the presidential campaign, *when the powers that govern our country would be forced to our assistance, or their party would go down in defeat.*

At a joint convention in Hazleton in the summer of 1900, delegates from throughout the hard-coal region sent Mitchell to New York to bring their grievances directly to the coal company presidents. Mitchell knocked on gilded doors that never opened and waited in ornate Wall Street anterooms for meetings that never took place. He asked friends of friends for letters of introduction, but all refused. Hearing a rumor that an Erie Railroad vice president lived at the Astor Hotel, he showed up unannounced. Who are you? the man said when he answered the door. I'm John Mitchell, president of the United Mine Workers of America. Can't be, said the Erie vice president. Mitchell would be an older man. No, it's me, I assure you. I may be young, he said, but I've been doing this all my life. The Erie man would not let Mitchell into his room, so they talked across the threshold. Mitchell explained that he was trying to avoid a strike and that his visit was a courtesy. I don't believe you fully appreciate the anger among the miners, he told the man. They are *not receiving proper wages,* and they are *not working under proper conditions.* They will strike if they don't get them. The Erie man, who didn't care, laughed and closed the door. The operators were united.

Under no circumstances, they told anyone who asked, *will we recognize the Mine Workers' Union.*

Mitchell returned to the coalfields to huddle with his union leaders. Despite the lack of a strike fund and no success organizing the eastern European miners, he called a region-wide strike in September 1900, which ended when the operators, using Gowen's old tactic, made a verbal promise to raise the wages by 10 percent and to listen to the miners' grievances. The union declared victory, which made John Mitchell a household name, but when the miners returned to work, they found conditions and wages unchanged. The operators evicted the most prominent union miners from company homes and blacklisted thousands more. They paid replacement miners lower wages by claiming that the agreement only covered existing miners. Foremen rejected every grievance brought by every committee of mine workers.

Mitchell refused to intervene when the miners complained, so each local confronted the coal companies on their own. Breaker boys refused to sort the coal that tumbled down the breaker's chutes. Union miners wore union buttons and refused to work with those who wouldn't. When foremen fired or suspended a union miner, for any reason, everyone walked off the job. Union locals throughout the coalfield established their own production quotas. No miner, they declared, should benefit at the expense of another miner. Every miner gets the same number of coal cars to load as every other miner, no exceptions. The teenage muledrivers enforced the new standard. *The runners have a rule,* a miner explained, *if an old man falls behind a strong man, the strong man has got to be held back, he has got to have an even number of cars on that division. They won't allow one chamber to have more cars than another chamber.* If a miner took more cars than allowed by the union, he was ejected from the local chapter. If he continued to fill more cars than permitted, a committee of miners paid him a visit and broke his tools.

If a foreman ordered a miner to violate a union rule, he laughed and said, *Johnnie Mitchell's my boss.*

The wildcat strikes spread and continued through 1901 and into 1902. The national leaders of the UMW finally agreed to meet in a joint convention in Shamokin in April 1902, where delegates established four principal demands. First, a 20 percent increase in wages for every miner, new or old. Second, a reduced workday—nine hours instead of ten—and no reduction in wages. Third, a demand to be paid by the weight of all coal mined, not the number of coal cars loaded. This was the primary demand. Underground coal cars were made of oak, but it was like they were made of live oak, always growing larger. Finally, they demanded a binding contract between the coal operators and the United Mine Workers of America. No more handshake agreements.

The convention sent fourteen miners to New York, but, as in 1900, the coal presidents refused to negotiate. We have a legal obligation to our shareholders, they explained, and this prohibits us from raising wages. There would be no coal companies without shareholders, they said. It is this investment that *renders the operations of our mines possible.* It may be true that the miners dig coal from the earth, the coal presidents conceded, but the shareholders own the earth. We cannot even recognize the union, much less negotiate with it, explained one president, for to do so would *destroy the corporation, for whose solvency and prosperity its officers were responsible.*

The National Civic Federation proposed a thirty-day truce, but when the parties reconvened in early May, the operators again refused to negotiate. We can't meet these wage demands, they said. We'd have to raise prices, and we'd lose market share to soft coal if we did, and this would mean that we would be unable to deliver the future we promised to our shareholders. We'll throw open our books if you don't believe us. The miners had no interest in the concerns of shareholders or the doctored books of the coal companies. The National Civic Federation proposed instead that smaller negotiating teams meet, but the coal companies refused, agreeing only to meet in sixty day's time.

On May 9, Mitchell called members of the anthracite district's executive board to Scranton's Carpenter's Hall, where they narrowly voted to declare a temporary work stoppage. After the vote, Mitchell stood on a chair in the middle of a crowd at the St. Charles hotel and told a crowd of miners and reporters that the work stoppage would not begin until May 12, which would give each local chapter a chance to meet and vote on whether to strike and then to select a delegate to represent it at the convention in Hazleton on May 14.

The mine workers understood the stakes. If they lost the strike and the coal presidents got their way, every future year would look like 1901, which was a year in which the mining of hard coal fractured the legs of 314 miners, snapped 97 arms in half, and burned nearly 245 miners to death. A year in which 219 miners suffered fractured skulls, 19 had their faces slashed, 72 had their teeth knocked clear out of their heads by props, mule kicks, or flying rocks. A year one miner lost an eye, six broke a jaw, sixty-two had a hand crushed, and forty-one had ribs not just broken but shattered to pieces and left floating in flesh. A year sixty-five hips and knees were crushed, ten collarbones were broken, sixty-nine ankles and feet were turned, twisted, and dislocated. A year 213 miners were committed to the poor house and 513 were crushed to death, drowned, or asphyxiated. A year nine or more miners were dragged dead from the mines or nearly dead every day. A year of misery for the miners and windfall profits for the mine owners. A year the coal companies sold more coal and made more money than in any previous year.

Mitchell counseled caution. *I am of the opinion*, he wrote to Mother Jones, *that it will be a fight to the end and our organization will either achieve a great triumph or it will be completely annihilated*. Some said, yes, it is true we will suffer in this fight, and we know that some will be blacklisted by the bosses and some will die at the hands of the police, but what else can we do? This is our one chance, and it might be our last. Let's finally make a stand, once and for all, on strike day in Hazleton.

CHAPTER THREE

ON STRIKE DAY IN HAZLETON

The cold front that arrived on the weekend before the Hazleton convention covered the blackened coalfields in a crystalline layer of frost that scattered light and muffled sound, leaving everything still and white, as if frozen in its own negative image. When the breaker whistles blew, calling the miners and breaker boys to work, only the firemen and pumpmen responded and only to keep the mines free of water in case the strike was called off. A few miners descended into the mines but only to carve an X on the top coal, marking breasts as theirs. They spent the rest of the day on the streets or in the saloons discussing their chances in the strike. Some of the eastern European miners took trains east, the start of a great return migration home. *They say they will go to Europe if a strike is declared*, reported the papers, *and remain there until the trouble is over.*

Some union delegates arrived in Hazleton as early as Monday, May 12, finding cheap lodging in the boarding houses. Dozens of reporters arrived and took rooms at the Valley Hotel, where they spent their days loitering in the lobby and listening for rumors. Mitchell arrived in Freeland, nine miles north of Hazleton, on Tuesday afternoon. He waved to a cheering crowd as he descended from the train to a four-horse carriage surrounded by a brigade of breaker boys standing in a ragged order. St. Anne's band played "Hail to the Chief" and paraded him through the streets. A thousand miners marched in military formation behind him. When they reached the Osborn House Hotel, Mitchell climbed up to a second-story balcony and gave a two-minute speech that took ten minutes to finish, what with all the cheering interrupting every sentence.

After the speech, he rode into Hazleton by buckboard and found a throng of miners—twenty thousand by some estimates—surrounding the Grand Opera House. Peddlers pushed handcarts through the crowd and sold UMW badges and colorful flags adorned with Mitchell's image. The delegates from the isolated mine patches and far-flung districts carried pasteboard boxes under their arms full of passenger pigeons. We plan to release them after the strike vote is made, they told curious reporters, to carry the news home. Marching bands paraded in from McAdoo and Freeland, like a festival day, as if the future had already been won.

The optimists among miners had reason to be confident. Every city everywhere used anthracite to fire boilers that ran engines that pumped groundwater. Silk mills and textile mills used it to power throwing machines. Hotels and apartment buildings burned it to run elevators and electric lights. The coal dealers had limited supplies on hand, a few weeks at the most, and no one knew what would happen when the coal ran out. The pessimists found reason to worry. What if the cities lift the prohibition against the burning of soft coal? We'll know we've lost the strike if we see the soot from *curling columns of black smoke* fill the skies. The largest factories had already begun buying soft coal. Only the launderers and house painters could see a silver lining in a thing like that.

The union leaders spent a restless night fending off the constant interruptions of the reporters, who doubted the miners could win. After all, *it was not arbitration the operators wanted,* the *New York Tribune* wrote, *but the life blood of the union.* Mitchell made no comment, but others had plenty to say. A representative of the Anthracite Coal Operators Association predicted the strike, if it came, would collapse in a matter of weeks. The merchants will cut them off and the operators will evict them from their homes, he said. They'll lose the sympathy of the public because their demands are unreasonable. If anything, the miners are overpaid. Overpaid? Yes, it's true, he said. The miners make anywhere from nine to fifteen dollars a day, he claimed. How could that be true? Most of them live in rough hovels crowded in miserable mine patches where coal dust piles up like snow drifts. Who would choose to live amid burning culm banks in fifteen-square-foot shanties made of sheet iron and scrounged materials perched on streets no wider than a miner's wingspan? Yes, it's true, he admitted. There are endless fields of squalid huts, but you don't understand them like we do. They live how they want. *As a matter of fact*, he proclaimed, *they won't live any other way.*

Tens of thousands of eastern European miners lived hand-to-mouth, that was true. They were refugees chased from their homelands by the crushing weight of taxes or the endless worry of conscription. They were Slovak peasants come to escape the forced assimilation of Hungarian nationalism. They were Catholic Polish peasants pushed from the eastern provinces by waves of German settlers. They were the Ruthenian sons of eastern Slavs from Galicia, sent to rescue families from the debt of dead cattle and failed harvests. Most worked for a dollar a day and lived on ten dollars a month. The bachelors bunked in barn-like boardinghouses for a dollar a month; the number of beds in a room determined by the number of beds a room could hold. These were collective affairs of twenty or more men run by a woman who charged extra for wash. They paid five dollars a month for huge communal dinners of stew meat, baking beans, and root vegetables. They saved their money and lived a what's-on-hand existence. They killed ducks for meat, set traps for game, gathered berries along railway lines, dug potatoes from farmers' lands. Most never bought a winter coat and suffered through winter in blue work overalls instead. Some few bought a cheap lot from a coal company and built a simple house from found materials. A railroad tie foundation, fence paling and driftwood cladding, scrap tin roof, a cheap stove for cooking and heating, scavenged coal taken from culm banks and cave-ins. They collected water from creeks or common wells, dug open-pit privies, burned their waste in huge firepits. They lived in worlds of their own collective making. They read their own newspapers in their own languages, built and attended their own churches, drank in their own saloons, pooled their money into their own building and loan associations, established their own secret, benevolent societies. *My people do not live in America*, explained a Greek Orthodox priest. *They live underneath America. America goes on over their heads.*

On Wednesday, May 14, the day the convention began, the delegates not already in Hazleton arrived on packed, early morning trains and trolleys. Those already in town ate boardinghouse breakfasts and then walked to the Opera House in small groups, finding the streets full of Polish and Lithuanian mine workers standing in tight groups or sitting on Broad Street's stone curbs, watching the marching bands parade down Broad Street. When the Opera House threw open its doors, the first delegates made a beeline to the upright piano on the far side of the stage. They sang union songs as miners in blue overalls or wool sack suits shuffled into the hall. They shook hands and said their hellos as they came in, filling row after row, moving to some kind of fraternal choreography. Thomas Duffy, the barrel-chested UMW district president, who came clean-shaven and in a wool vest, climbed to a stage festooned with Fourth of July buntings and UMW flags and called the convention to order. I need a nomination for a temporary chairman, he hollered, and a thousand voices shouted John Mitchell!

Mitchell, sitting stageside, stood when his name was called. He took his hat from his head and ran a hand through short, black hair, then climbed to the stage as the miners roared their approval. When he got to the center of the stage, he turned toward the miners and stretched his arms out wide, quieting their applause. His round face flushed red against his starched white collar. Gentlemen, he said, speaking loudly so the delegates in the balcony could hear him, your meeting here today is fraught with great responsibility. *You are going to decide the most important movement in the history of the entire anthracite coal industry, if not in the labor movement of the world.* The time for speeches will be later, he said. For now, our job is to elect a convention secretary and a sergeant-at-arms. In the days prior to the convention, rumors had circulated that the coal operators planned to infiltrate the convention, as they always did. We'll need a doorkeeper posted at the entryway and a credentials committee, he said, so that only official delegates can gain entry. A miner named Edwards shouted his agreement. *At Shamokin we had people in our convention who were not delegates.* A round of nominations were made and then a quick straw vote was taken. When three men were selected for the job, Mitchell asked for a motion to adjourn until 1:30 p.m. so the committee could make an official roster of delegates. The miners filed out of the Opera House in twos and threes. Some headed to the Crystal Palace Lunch Parlor or the counter at Wear's, where they found oxtail soup and brook trout on lunch special. A few dozen skipped lunch and instead followed Mitchell out the door and past the stables to the Valley Hotel half a block away, where they formed a line outside his door, hoping for a private audience.

When the convention reconvened, the credentials committee sent word that it needed more time to finalize the delegate roster. To kill the time, four miners took to the stage to lead the theater in a rendition of the Welsh labor song "Comrades in Arms."

You are my shipmates as we sail through the storm
You are my partners-in-crime, and you always want more
You're my reminder, when the going gets tough
You are my comrades in arms, and we'll never give up.

Applause filled the hall when they finished. Someone whispered in Mitchell's ear. The credentials committee needs more time, he announced. A Plymouth delegate offered to fill the time with a live demonstration on the proper use of squibs for the safe firing of black powder. The miners murmured their agreement, and the man passed out bags of squibs row by row, making a show of being careful as he did it. Too many hands get mangled and too many eyes get blown out from the improper use of squibs, he said. He spent the next hour demonstrating how to handle them safely, what to do when they got wet, and the safest way to insert them into the powder cartridges, finishing his presentation just as the three-man credentials committee finally reentered the hall. They took the stage and spent the next hour taking turns reading the names of confirmed delegates from each district. When they finished, dozens of men came to the stage to say they hadn't heard their names. I guess we need more time to finalize our report on credentials, they conceded. Can't we just come up with a temporary password to control access to the hall until the roster is ready? asked a delegate named Gildea. It'd be easier to *just use the old password*, said another man. Mitchell agreed but others objected. *Half of us have forgotten it.* Let's just be patient and wait for the final credentials. No, said another delegate, making a motion that they just vouch for each other. No, that won't work either, said a delegate named Edwards. The only man who can vouch for me is my district secretary and he's on the credentials committee. A few frustrated delegates took out pocket watches, showed them around, raised their eyebrows and shook their heads. Some miners took to their feet to talk in the aisles, while others smoked in the lobby so they could talk above a whisper.

A pickpocket worked his way through the crowd, taking advantage of the delay. The Shamokin miner Nelson Yoder got clipped for eleven dollars and didn't even notice until lunch. The Reverend Father T. R. Watkins, the Scranton preacher who'd quit God to mine coal, got touched for ten dollars and even lost his train ticket home. The Lansford delegate Cavanaugh got knuckled for forty-seven dollars and his comrade James Dick, also from Lansford, had eleven lifted from him. Either from the pickpocket or the meandering discussion, some delegates had had enough, Wasn't this the work of the credentials committee? *Didn't they just establish a man's right to sit here?* asked one delegate. It's clear the delegates present are not in shape to do business, said another. We're wasting valuable time and getting into such *a tangle over nothing.* Others seemed unconcerned. We expected this, they said. Let's just wait until we get the final credentials report. Mitchell, impatient too, ended the discussion. *Gentlemen, the password each delegate will give to the Sergeant-at-Arms is Patience.* Without missing a beat, a delegate named Llewellyn said he thought it would be *up to the chair to be patient. He'll need patience more than the delegates.*

The afternoon was given over to announcements. Each announcement was introduced as the last but was always followed by another. The men who predicted a one-day convention caught I-told-you-so looks from the miners who predicted two. A union officer cautioned the delegates about the dance planned for that night at Brennan's Hall in Polish McAdoo. It's a big affair, a regular thing. He'd heard some delegates were planning to attend that night, but since the orchestra at the event was no friend to the miners, it was decided no one should go. They're *partly on the unfair list,* he explained. Mitchell read a letter from a local regalia-making company in Hazleton, announcing that they'd gifted shiny new UMW badges to every delegate. Pick one up on your way out of the hall, he said, finally calling an end to the first day of the convention. We reconvene tomorrow at 9:00 a.m., he said, as the miners bottlenecked their way down the aisles and out onto the street, where they were immediately besieged by reporters. No, they told anyone who asked, we didn't get a chance to discuss the strike today, but we hope to tomorrow. The younger miners caught a trolley into McAdoo. Some visited saloons. Mitchell was mobbed as he made his way back to the hotel. The streets remained crowded late into the night, though locals remarked how quiet everything seemed. These miners are earnest, all agreed.

Reporters began knocking on Mitchell's door by seven on Thursday morning. What about the miners? they asked. Do you have a sense of what they're thinking? A majority of the delegates seem to favor a strike, he told them. Outside, the day dawned windy and warmer. A group of breaker boys snuck through a hole in the fence that surrounded the house of John Markle, the rich coal operator, and spent the day loafing on his front porch. Hundreds of people loitered on the street between Vine and Church, smoking pipes and waiting for news from the convention. A hum of anticipation filled the lobby of the Valley Hotel. When a stranger walked through with a Pittsburgh paper sticking out of his coat pocket, reporters ran after him, yelling questions. Are you with the bituminous men? There were more than thirty thousand soft coal miners in western Pennsylvania. Will they strike too? A young Hazleton man loud-talked his way around the lobby telling everyone within earshot he had inside information. He offered four-to-one odds that the miners wouldn't strike, but he found no takers.

The Opera House was full by 9:00 a.m., all except for Mitchell, who'd left his hotel room with plenty of time to spare but couldn't *walk ten paces without someone stopping him, asking him questions, encouraging him, pleading with him, reminding him of this or that fact he might have forgotten*. Mitchell politely listened to every appeal, promised to consider their concerns, took note of every suggestion, and was half an hour late to the convention because of it.

He entered the hall to applause and walked directly to the stage where he brought the convention to order. He took a telegram out of the inside pocket of his coat jacket and read it aloud while a few smokers straggled in from the lobby. The Iowa miners wish us success, he said, holding up the telegram. *They pledge to us their fraternal feelings.* The credentials committee worked all night and finally had a roster for the convention. The 359 union locals of the anthracite coalfields had sent 627 delegates to Hazleton where they would cast 979 votes. Mitchell stepped back to the stage. *Gentlemen, I presume the time has come for you to determine what action you intend to take. Before doing so you will doubtless want a report of the special committee who represent you in the hearings in New York City.* He launched into a timeline of everything they'd done since the April convention in Shamokin. He described how the National Civic Federation had tried to use its *good offices to bring about a peaceful solution.* He mentioned how the thirty-day truce and follow-up meeting had come to nothing. At every step, he told them, the operators refused *to concede anything.* Their only offer was to let us examine their books, which, he said, we declined to do. A subcommittee met with George Baer and two other coal presidents, but that ended without an agreement, like all the other meetings. Their last proposal was to meet again in sixty days. Last week, in Scranton, we debated how to proceed. Though *the committee was not unanimous in its opinion as to the time the strike should be inaugurated*, it did *decide to order a temporary suspension of work and to call this convention. They wished to allow the miners to determine for themselves what course they desired to pursue.* It's up to you now, he said, imploring them to set all other concerns aside. Don't make this about the man who makes the argument, instead give every delegate your *careful attention.* Give every miner *a full and respectful hearing today.*

The question now before the house is: *Shall the temporary suspension be made permanent? Will you declare for a strike now? Will you defer the time of strike, or what will you do about it?* He asked for a motion.

Half-dead Jimmy Gallagher's son stood up. *I came here instructed to vote for a strike or to continue the suspension if no concessions had been gained. That is the feeling of the people in my local. We can see very plainly that no concessions will be granted.* He reminded them that some locals were already out on strike. We won't have a union *if we desert the men who have been out on strike for the past three months.* They expected something from us at the Shamokin convention in April, but we didn't deliver it. We can now. No more delay. I claim that it *is the proper time to strike. If we defer the commencement of our strike until six months from today* the operators will have time to prepare. *I think that must be plain to all of you.* This isn't a fight over wages and working conditions. We know what's at stake here. It's *not the paltry sum of an increase of 10 percent in your wages that the operators care so much about. No, that's not what they're fighting you for. They want to get your organization out of existence so that they will have no more trouble with you.* They don't want to meet committees of miners every sixty days. That's just a ploy. *They want to have you in such a condition that they can treat with you as they have been doing for the last fifteen years.* Let's finally settle our own troubles.

As soon as Gallagher finished, another delegate stood up and objected to everything he said, complaining that *the time for speech-making had passed.* We've all made up our minds, he said. Most of our locals sent us here with instructions on how to vote. We're only messengers sent to carry the sentiment of our locals. My local wants the suspension continued and efforts likes those of the last few months to continue. He made a motion to extend the temporary suspension, which was quickly seconded.

A delegate named Quigley stood to oppose the motion. If it's true that most of us come with instructions, what's the point of debating? The decision's already been made. Let's find out where we all stand. He called for a roll call vote. What's the point of that? asked a delegate named Davis. Let's just vote on whether to strike or not. That's the question. *I don't see that we can do anything else.* I say we strike. If we don't, we're back in the *same position we were in thirteen weeks ago.* He reminded the delegates that his local has been on strike since February. We're ready to fight for this organization or go down with it. The operators *have four or five million tons of coal* in reserve, but *that is not enough to run the Atlantic steamers and supply factories for a week.* Delay strengthens their hands. Now's our chance, not later.

A cautious faction opposed the strike. The first among them to speak was a delegate named Picton, who told the convention not to run away with the idea that he's some conservative miner who refuses to confront the operators. We just want fair play, he said. We want to be able to have a voice in all this, some influence. *I'm voting as instructed, but I have discretion,* he promised. Mitchell interrupted him. Everyone will have a vote. Let's not waste time debating whether we'll be heard or not. *Focus on the motion, no one's shut out.*

A delegate named John Taylor stood to say he had no discretion at all. I've been sent to Hazleton to vote for a strike unless *it can be shown that concessions have been made.* That's the question we have to answer. I don't see any concessions made by the operators. Delegate Llewellyn agreed. And it's not for a lack of trying, he said. We've got the most conservative labor leaders *the world has ever seen* and what has that gotten us? *We've gone on our knees to the operators. Shall we go on our knees again? While we were on our knees begging they turned their backs on us and spurned us.* There have been no concessions at all.

A delegate named Watkins, who said he'd spent the last twenty-two years buried in the earth mining coal directly beneath their feet, said he'd *attended a great many conventions* and had *seen a great many strikes* and the one thing he'd learned is that the difficulty is not in calling a strike or in timing it right, the key is sustaining it. We should require a two-thirds vote to call a strike. That might *help the weak-kneed brothers in the organization. I know from experience that there are always weak-kneed brothers who need to be encouraged.*

The specter of weak-kneed brothers brought Neil M'Kechnie to his feet. I've heard this talk about weak-kneed brothers, he said. Let's hear from them. *Who opposes this?* So far I have not heard much from those who oppose it here, he said, looking around the hall at the miners looking back at him. *I would like to hear from someone who is opposed to striking under the conditions we are now suffering from under our employers.* He stopped, held up a hand, said no, that's not right. They're not our employers. *I might say our lords and kings. I think we really have more lords and kings here than they have in Europe. I've been a miner my whole life. I've worked in all kinds of mines from gold to salt mines and have never in the thirty-eight years of my mining experience been treated worse than we're being treated in the Wyoming Valley at the present time.* I've been with every union organized in these parts, he said. The old WBA and all the rest. This is the worst we've had it. *Think of less than five thousand people in the United States owning sixteen billion dollars of the wealth, and there are nearly a hundred million of us. For 364 days of the year, we work for them, and the 365th we go and vote to put them in power to continue this state of affairs?*

M'Kechnie's speech had the effect of sharpening the debate and making opposition to the strike a sign of weakness or appeasement, which brought a delegate named Echersly to his feet. We're not scared of striking, he explained. This isn't just a question whether to go out on strike or not, he said. Despite what some think, our chances of success are absolutely a question of timing. *I think the first of September would be a better time to strike than the present* when the coming of winter would work on our behalf. Another delegate agreed, saying it would give the union a chance to build up a strike fund. *If we have a strike that will last for six months, where are we to get relief?*

Let's not get ahead of ourselves, cautioned a delegate named Gilchrist. Those sent here with instructions to strike were told to vote for the strike unless the operators made concessions. Didn't the operators agree to meet with us every sixty days? Isn't that a concession? he asked. *Our local would be satisfied with that. We must not expect too much all at one time.* His comment drew an angry response from the Delegate John Reap. You call that a concession? he asked sarcastically. It sounds more like fear, like a way to talk yourself out of doing the right thing. Look at all we've done. We offered to arbitrate. We conceded to them on our wage demands. What have they done? They've offered nothing. *I have been in three or four strikes and was not prepared to meet any of them* because there's no preparing for a thing like this. *I cannot say positively that I am the owner of ten dollars* but that doesn't matter. The time to strike is now. *There is no other honorable course left to us.*

Delegates were now lining up to speak, and talking louder when they did. *I'm willing to fight and die under Mitchell,* said one. Exactly, said a delegate named Lewis. *What is there left for us to do? We sent these men to New York, and they did everything in their power to get the corporations to grant concessions and avert this miserable strike.* We'll suffer in this strike, we'll pay the price, but that's no reason to hesitate. *What people on the face of the earth ever bettered their condition without paying a price?* I've been thrown out of work in the dead of winter before. I know suffering. *I am a soldier. I fought to free the Black slaves of the South, and now I am ready to fight to the death before I shall go back into white slavery here in Pennsylvania.*

An uncertain delegate offered to vote for the strike but only if he got a guarantee in return. We've been here before, and we've lost. What makes this moment any different? *If anyone can convince me that we shall win I shall hold my hand up for a strike.* For one thing, replied Delegate J. M. Loeffler, our best chance is now. It would be the operators who *would be better off later, not us.* They have little coal in reserve, *but they'll have a good supply if we postpone this for a month or two.* Each comment drew cheers from those who agreed with it and murmurs from those opposed it. The back and forth continued until Peter McHale stood up. What is this, a debating society? *The time for deliberation, consideration and investigation by the miners is done.* We're just digging in at this point. We should vote. Our leaders have won for us a great victory already. *They have proved to the world that we are in the right. The time has come for us to go ahead. We all know the false hopes with which the operators have tried to fill our souls.* That so-called thirty-day truce was one of them. *We know we are right, let's go ahead.* Another delegate agreed. What's the point of discussing whether to fight when we all know *the fight has already begun.* We're already in the ring. What boxer enters a ring and throws no punches? If you think conditions are not right, work to change them. If you think we need a stronger organization, work to make it stronger. But don't fool yourself. We're already in a fight. The only thing yet to do is fight back. And don't forget, said the delegate Dempsey, it's not like we asked for this. *The challenge has been forced on us.* He dismissed the arguments of the delegates who saw concessions everywhere they looked. Should we consider it a concession that they bought our leaders lunch in New York? Are we to consider it a concession that their refusal to arbitrate was somehow an acknowledgment that something needed arbitrating? Don't pretend we have any choice here. There's no going back to the mines at this point. The operators are on a war footing now and if we return, they *will turn their guns on the Local officers. Then when we want to strike there will be no organization to strike with.* He dismissed the idea that their demands had gone too far. Some who oppose this strike, he said, call the demands we agreed to in Shamokin unreasonable, radical even. What's radical about demanding back *one penny of the millions of dollars that have been stolen from us and from our fathers?* Is that unreasonable? And don't forget, we have allies in this struggle. *This is not only our fight. It is the fight of 4,500,000 men who are affiliated with the American Federation of Labor.*

Stolen from us, yes! insisted Delegate Carne. At my local, when we voted on the strike, we talked about *the millions of tons of coal that have been stolen from the miners in years gone by.* Who would deny this? *I for one will not yield one inch in the struggle before us.* They take from us and will not concede on anything. *They have had the reins in their hands so long and have pulled us hither and thither at their own will so long. They will not likely give that up now.* What have we been doing these past years if not readying ourselves for this moment? I, like so many of you, am *foot-sore* from all the organizing and fighting I have done. My local instructed me to vote to strike *regardless of anything and everything because they say they have put up with everything that is bearable. They have given the companies more than we could afford to give them.* If we back down now, it only gets worse. *How long will it be before some of us will have to travel the continent blacklisted by the operators?* Condemned to be labor's vanquished vagabonds. The last words they said to me when they sent me here as a delegate was, *If you don't vote to strike don't come back here.* He paused, calmed his voice, and appealed to those who opposed the strike. You conservative men, fine, be conservative. It is right to have your arguments, but we must be unanimous here. You all know *they have robbed us* of what's ours. This is our best chance to take it back. We might not win this, *but I'd rather go down to my grave fighting a brave fight than to again wander over the country blacklisted.* What do we have to lose that we haven't already lost? *If we must go down, let's go down fighting.*

A motion to end debate was made and seconded. Mitchell called all those who supported the motion to say yea. A thunder of yeas filled the hall. All those opposed, say nay. The roar of nays sounded equal to the ayes. Mitchell smiled and shook his head, looking to the convention secretary for help. What should we do? Dozens of delegates shouted roll call. T. D. Nichols waved them off. That'll just take longer than letting the debate take its course. Continue, he said.

Delegates who wanted to fight but feared the outcome sought reassurance. A delegate named Gallagher said he didn't disagree with the arguments to strike. It's not the operators I fear, he explained. It's our will to fight that I doubt. Some miners are doing better than others, he said. *I have seen the day in the anthracite coal region when the people above struck and the people below went on working, and I have seen the people below strike and the people above keep on working, and thus the market was supplied with coal and the strikes failed in nearly every case. How strong are we, really? How many of our 144,000 men attends their locals or pays their dues regularly?* We need help to win this. We need the soft coal miners to strike with us. If they don't, the soft coal will replace anthracite, and we'll lose. Mitchell can tell us, someone shouted. A motion was made and quickly seconded to have Mitchell speak to the strength of the union, but Mitchell refused. *That motion will not be entertained at this time,* he said.

The miners knew their leaders were cautious. Many assumed they opposed the strike, but none had yet made their views clear. George Hartlein, the prominent District 9 secretary, finally rose to his feet. Gentlemen, he said, the operators *will come out in the public press, which they own or control, and they will say they offered to submit the books of the companies to you, and the public will say, the miners have refused to examine the books.* What are they afraid of? If we strike, we will have public opinion against us, and *you cannot win without public opinion.* He claimed the operatives had, in fact, made concessions. Consider all we've accomplished since 1900, he said. *The supreme head of the anthracite coal operators has meekly submitted to meet Mr. Mitchell, Mr. Fahy and Mr. Nichols and those who accompanied them, and talked their differences over, not alone for one day, but for three days.* They have invited us to talk. This is not something they've done before. *Concessions have been made. The public of New York have been told by some of the greatest financiers of New York that the anthracite miners have deeply impressed them with the honesty of their intentions. If you go into a fight you will open up sores that will take years and years to heal over.* They agreed to meet us every sixty days, he said. *Is that a step backward?* You sent Mitchell to meet with them. *They have done that.* This is progress, and because of it, and with all their concessions, we are *not at this time justified in going into a strike.* Hartlein's speech angered nearly every delegate. Those who supported the strike dismissed his wishful thinking as Siney-like. Those who opposed the strike wished he'd said it a hell of a lot earlier. Why didn't you say all this before the locals held their votes? The hall erupted in shouts of competing complaints to Hartlein. Mitchell silenced them, reminding them that Hartlein had the right to say whatever he wanted to say, whenever he wanted.

Delegate Bernard Duffy stood up and told Hartlein he was wrong about public opinion. No one alive would say we're not justified. Who cares that we refused to examine their books. Who could object to that? No one could make heads or tails out of them anyway. A delegate named Jones agreed, dismissing the concerns about timing. Who can say whether we're ready or not? No one denies the conditions could be better, but why let that determine when we fight? This brought Delegate Dempsey to his feet, shaking his head. What a thing to dismiss, he said. If we can't even explain to ourselves how to win, why would we go out on strike? The point of a strike isn't to successfully go out on strike, it's to win what can't be won without a strike. We ought to be certain we can win. *I do not believe it is good policy to strike now because your demands have been ignored. It's all very well to stand up here and tell of the demands you have made, of the treatment you have received, grow patriotic and yell for a strike. I want you to get up here and show me the ammunition you're going to fight with.* We can lay down our tools and shut down the mines, but what then? How will we take care of nearly 150,000 men when we have no strike fund? We need to determine what we need to win this. As I see it, the only way to win is to make it a general strike of every coal miner in the country. *Let it be from ocean to ocean and tie up the markets right.* If we strike now, just us and us alone, how will you stand it? *Where will you get aid if you strike?* Don't get me wrong. *If we vote to strike, I will be there with you. I will fight as long as any other man will fight with me.* I am not opposed to striking. I am opposed to losing. Delegate Clauser told the convention the union was stronger than some think. *There was not a single union man in my place last time. Now they're all with the union. In the meeting that selected me as the delegate to this convention, the members went wild.* They're ready to fight, and they won't waver.

A line of delegates waited to talk, but Mitchell adjourned the convention until 1:30 p.m. The miners argued their way out of the hall and spilled out onto Broad Street. Waiting reporters ran up to those they recognized. Yes, we're still debating, the delegates said. Yes, there seems to be great sentiment to strike, but there's no telling how this will turn out. No, they said, Mitchell hasn't addressed the convention. We expect he will when we reconvene, they said. After the break, as the delegates returned, they mingled in groups at the edges of the stage and in the aisles. Some smoked in the lobby, reluctant to return, but then a delegate poked his head out to say that De Silva was about to speak. Finally, the trusted De Silva, Civil War hero. If anyone other than Mitchell could sway the vote, it would be De Silva.

He began by admitting he was more uncertain now than before the convention. The delegates who oppose the strike say it will destroy our organization if we strike, and the delegates who support it say it will destroy our organization if we don't strike. He told the delegates he felt that moment the way he felt at the Battle of Fredericksburg, when twenty thousand men died in battle. *From morning till night one line after another of Union soldiers were hurled against the heights of Fredericksburg. From ten o'clock in the morning until darkness fell, one line after another went up there to meet what they knew was certain defeat. And the last line that went up that day, the line I had the honor of being in, advanced further up the hill and closer to the Rebel lines than any other line of the day. And yet we were shattered more because we were closer and met the fate of the others. We retreated, but by half past four next morning those same lines faced the same enemy, just as willing to be sacrificed as they had been the day before.* Those soldiers didn't ask for guarantees. They knew there is only the will to fight or the lack of it. Only *when this organization can make up its mind that it will face the enemy, and if it gets whipped retreat, reorganize, and come up again, will we have gained a victory, a victory greater than we have ever gained before.* Victory is the condition of living despite defeat. It is *the ability to stand defeat and come up and fight another day.* Many of you have told us your instructions, so I'll tell mine. *Our local voted for a strike, there being a majority of only one for it. After this vote was taken, and as the majority was so small, they considered it better to leave the delegates to their own judgement.* I visited other locals to find out how they bore this great responsibility. At one, *an old miner got up and said, Brother, can you tell us how this will come out if we strike? I considered a moment and said, Brothers, I am pretty well advanced in years. I have not very many years left, but I believe I would be willing to sacrifice one of those years if I could answer that question. That is exactly the way I feel today.* Here is what I know for sure: *We have postponed action now for forty-five days and have learned that that is not the best thing to do. We all feel that it has placed us at a disadvantage. I think if I have learned anything it is that that would not be the safest way of opening a fight.* I've heard Brother Mitchell say that every labor leader gets crucified in the end. He accepts it as his fate. Do you? *If we go into this strike, we must understand that every man must go in on his own bottom.* There's no way to know what to expect. You can only rely on your comrade if you first rely on yourself. *You must go in with the determination to stand, and stand until you win, and that without the assistance of anybody.* I can't tell anyone how to vote. Just be clear about what you choose and know well what it takes to win when you choose it.

De Silva took his seat and the delegates who followed him no longer talked about the wisdom of striking but instead about the character of the fight already underway. One said his local had been on strike for ten months already, and the miners there *are just as staunch today as the day they went out.* De Silva is right, said the man. This is not about preparing for a strike or predicting its outcome. *I had not a second loaf of bread in my house in 1900, yet I had a family to support. I came out with the rest and did not ask for assistance. All we have to do is put on our armor, buckle it tight, and say that we defy the coal barons of Pennsylvania.* A delegate named Sweeney said, Yes, but this isn't Fredericksburg. What about our lukewarm members who don't pay their dues? T. D. Nichols, good friend to Mother Jones, jumped to his feet to answer. I was hesitant to speak, he said, what with *so much talk in the papers about Nichols being bull-headed for a fight and all that,* but I object to Sweeney's comments here. I say we enter this fight and win it. Some here *speak of this organization as if it's something nailed together, tied with strings, or bound together with bands.* I don't recognize that. We act together. We've seen how the capitalists act together and we've seen what it does for them. There's nothing tangible we can point to that can guarantee our victory. We have *only the resolution of the men to act together. We know that to leave the union, to withdraw ourselves from each other, would be to place us wholly at the mercy of the other fellow. I think the anthracite miner has learned he dare not separate himself from the others and leave this organization.* We can worry about our every disadvantage. We can *worry that the companies are watching us; that they will find out what we have done in this convention and what we hope to do later on.* It's true. They know everything we do and plan to do. *We cannot keep our intentions secret from them.* If we say we plan to wait until the fall, they'll know it as soon as we say it, and they'll prepare for it. But that's paying attention to the wrong thing. *We're not hopeless.* You want to know how we win? *We all fall in line and that's how we'll win.*

More delegates who opposed the strike rose to their feet and poured out their fears. We're not strong enough financially, one said. Our spirit is not determined enough, said another. My local has no money saved up, added a third. This fight hasn't even started yet and already *we have hungry wolves at our door.* Imagine what it will be like months into this strike in the middle of winter, one said. If we lose, *someone will have to organize our children because we won't be around.*

There was no escaping the fear. To work was to be stalked by *a continuous spectacle of death and injury.* To go out on strike was to live in the shadow of the blacklist. Let's choose to fight, said a delegate named Matti. We don't have much, but don't we have our fists? Let's use them. Some say if we go on strike we cannot live. They talk of the assistance we will need. *To hear them one would think they could not live an hour, that they would die right away,* but don't give in to the fear. We are stronger than we think. A delegate named Spaide stood up. If you are paralyzed by fear, take comfort in knowing that the die has already been cast. The choice has been taken from you, and there is a freedom in that. It's time to use your fists. When my local voted to strike, the foreman forced the engineers and firemen and pumpmen to take a side. They did it. No handwringing. They set their fear aside and told the boss to a man that they would stand by us. *Then they were suspended until further notice.* If you can't fight for yourself, fight for them. And take comfort in knowing that your comrades are already fighting for you. Delegate Clark stood as if called to attention and declared that he was ready for the fight. Just let me know when I'll finally get the chance. A groundswell of strike sentiment rose, mixing with the cigar smoke wafting up to the balcony. Three delegates in succession said similar things. Another motion was made to end debate. It was seconded. Finally, the time to vote had arrived.

This was the moment Mitchell had been waiting for. He stood and faced the miners. After the convention, in letters he would write to friends and comrades, he would explain his reasons for opposing the strike. It wasn't because, like Siney, he saw friends where enemies lurked. He had no faith in the market. He was conservative, true, but not conservative in the way the coal presidents were. His conservatism was not a dream-politics of personal wealth. He was a coal miner, which meant his life had been a working life of accidents barely avoided and explosions narrowly escaped, a life of collapsing roofs and fizzled squibs, a life digging his own grave. When coal presidents lose, they lose money. When coal miners lose, they die. He began by thanking them for letting him serve them. It has been a privilege, *a treasure,* to have *held your confidence.* For that I owe you my honest opinion. *Don't violate your oath.* I've thought about nothing else. I've dreamed about it. *It has never been absent from my mind.* It is not for me to tell you what to do. It is true that the president of the United Mine Workers of America can reject a strike vote, but I won't do that. You were sent here to cast a vote. Do it. *Vote in accordance with those instructions no matter what.*

I will tell you honestly what I think. They want to destroy this union, like they've destroyed every union before us. What will happen to us if they win again? *When once the miners met a crushing defeat, it took years and years for them to recover from that defeat and again organize and renew the struggle.* The mine owners once ignored us, but they can't any longer. They once wouldn't even meet with me, now they open their offices to us. They once *sat in their beautiful homes* and declared they'd never meet with the officers of the United Mine Workers of America, but they do it now, don't they? Didn't they call us ruffians and cutthroats, Molly Maguires? *I am not one of those who believe the Molly Maguires were cut-throats at all*, but they do. And you know what they do to Molly Maguires. But now they know who we are. Think of the people who once condemned us but now offer support. The Civic Federation, bishops, senators. They say publicly we have the better case.

Mitchell walked to the side of the stage and grabbed a stack of papers from a table and held them aloft. I have letters I can show you from coal presidents who say they will recognize the union. They don't do it the way you want them to do it, but still, *they will receive committees and agree to take up for adjudication any grievances the men have*. I know you'll say that this is a small step forward. True, but doesn't every step matter? *Every indication is that progress is being made.* If it were my choice, I'd *agree to work for these wages and these conditions for one year*, but it is not my choice, or any one miner. It's our decision to make. I only ask that you keep one question at the forefront of your mind. *Is it better to go on improving your conditions, little by little, or to risk everything in one great fight? If I were sure, or if I believed that the fight could be won in a reasonable length of time, I should be willing to take that risk and advise you to take it. But gentlemen, this strike is not going to be for what they have offered and what you demand. This fight will be to the finish. It will be either a grand and mighty triumph for you, or it will throw you back to where you were before the strike of 1900. Back when a foreman could come around in the morning and send as many of the men home as he saw fit, and the men dared not resent it. It was their custom then to dock the miners as much and as often as they wanted to, and the men, because of their lack of organization, were unable to resist it.* I don't say you should be satisfied. *I will never be contented myself, and I hope to God you will not be either.* Rather I say that *I believe we can work this problem out by the methods we have been pursing.* He read a telegram from Ralph Easley, the head of the National Civic Federation, describing all the things the Federation proposed to do on the miners' behalf. He apologized for speaking for so long and then concluded by promising to fight beside them if they voted to strike. *It will be a long strike. It will be a strike to the finish.* He paused and took a deep breath, choosing his words carefully. But gentlemen, you must know that *if a strike must come, I shall be here to give you whatever assistance I have it in my power to give.* And then he took his seat.

A motion was made and seconded to close debate. The secretary prepared the rosters and readied the roll call. A district president passed a hat for the survivors of Lattimer and collected $42.33. Mitchell stood back up and said it was time. He asked them to stay in the hall during and after the roll call. After Delegate Ruscavage translated the instructions into Polish, the convention secretary began calling out names, one after the other. They stood when their names were called and shouted out their answer. When they were done, 461 delegates voted to strike and 349 voted to keep working. To a steady applause, Mitchell declared the motion carried, which grew louder when Delegate Thomas motioned to make the vote unanimous.

As the miners made their way to the doors, they were stopped by a delegate from Wilberton who loudly asked, but what about the police? *I was instructed to ask if the miners will be allowed to guard the operators' property. Our superintendent said he would rather have United Mine Workers guard the property than to have deputies guard it.* We should decide this before we adjourn. Some delegates waved it off as unimportant. Others argued that strikers should be permitted to take up positions as police and watchmen. It's up to them. Better us than the cut-throats and riffraff they'll ship from Philadelphia. Some have already taken up positions as police, said one delegate. They hold Coal and Iron Police commissions but *are heart and soul with us.* Some agreed to the idea of serving as watchmen but drew a line at police. *It'd show good spirit on the part of this convention to leave our brothers to act as watchmen,* one said, but serving as Coal and Iron Police makes no sense. *Why would we guard scabs who were taking our places?* But a loud minority drew a brighter line. We shouldn't allow this, they warned. No striker should serve as a watchman or for the Coal and Iron Police. Consider what that would mean. If anything does happen, it'll be the strikers who do it, and then the strikers-as-cops will be ordered to *turn their guns on their fellow United Mine Workers.*

The specter of Lattimer hung over the convention hall, complicating the debate. Remember Lattimer had become the watchwords for the Hazleton convention delegates. Every delegate who supported the proposal to let strikers serve as police raised its specter. If we had done this at Lattimer, a prominent union leader argued, *I don't think these men would have been killed, shot down on the highways.* If we fill these positions, *we can prevent thugs and cut-throats from Pittsburgh and Chicago and New York from coming in here and committing murder. You men have consciences and will not do wrong when sworn in as deputies, but the men that will end up here if you do not take the places will be thugs from the large cities, and they will be without consciences, and will do whatever they are ordered to do.*

Delegate after delegate rose in agreement. This will keep the Pinkertons out, said one. True, said the legendary John Fahy, the organizer of the first local UMW chapter in the anthracite fields. He argued that it was the man behind the badge that was the problem, not the badge. The law doesn't require that *police murder on command. I would rather have a Winchester in the hands of a man I thought was a sympathizer than in the hands of one who was anxious to shoot me down.* A vocal minority argued against the proposal. There's a reason they hire cutthroats to work as cops. *If you think the operators are so much inclined towards the United Mine Workers that they would trust their property to us, why do they not make concession to the workers that would prevent the necessity of having watchmen at all?* A majority of delegates ignored these warnings and voted instead to allow the strikers to serve as police.

With their business done, the delegates nominated Mitchell to make the announcement on the street. When he emerged from the Opera House, someone dragged over a box for him to stand on. He raised his hands to silence the reporters' questions. The delegates have voted unanimously to strike, he said. Some reporters shouted questions but most just turned and raced to the telegraph wires and hotel phone bank. A band appeared. A carriage rode up. Mitchell was hoisted into it and paraded through Hazleton. Pigeons filled the sky.

A reporter asked a worried-looking miner from Jeddo why he wasn't celebrating. *I have a wife and six children. I would like to stand by the union and get the concessions, but I don't see how I can let the little ones starve. We have only provisions for a week at the outside, and I can't see what I can do to earn a living except to work in the mines.*

The coal companies drew fire from their boilers, hoisted mules from the mines, and sent their coal cars west to the bituminous coalfields. The railroads furloughed the crews that hauled the coal. The yardmasters were laid off and the clerks who refused to serve as Coal and Iron Police were fired. Rumors began to spread that the union would call out the pumpmen and drown the mines with water. Once the mines are destroyed, they plan to declare a general strike and order every miner in the United States—nearly 500,000 of them—out of the mines. Panic set in. Old men presented themselves at the poor houses asking to be admitted. Newspapers warned of a coal famine. Coal dealers raised the price of coal by a dollar and threatened more. Cities cut power in the evenings to save on fuel. The silk factories shut down and laid off the mill girls. Labor agents appeared at the train depots and offered striking miners jobs out west at four times the wages paid in Pennsylvania, easy hours too, and company houses fit for the whole family. Mitchell warned the miners to stay clear of them, but some accepted their offers. Thousands of Irish and Welsh miners boarded westbound trains for temporary jobs and days later found themselves in distant scab camps guarded by armed deputies. The Polish, Slovak, and Lithuanian miners from Shenandoah and Duryea took their money out of banks and building and loans and boarded trains for New York, where they booked steamships back to Europe. A thousand abandoned Mahanoy City on May 19. Two thousand left Shenandoah the same day. Two weeks after the Hazleton convention, 25,000 miners had returned to Europe to wait out the strike.

The miners who lived in boarding houses had no income for rent, so they set up tent encampments near Blairsville and hoped for a quick resolution. The companies threatened to evict the remaining miners from the company shanties, but few believed them. With what army? Those who remained planned to survive on backyard gardens, store credit, and scavenged coal. Women picked huckleberries and sold them door to door for five cents a quart. By July, a Schuylkill shipper was buying them all up and shipping fifteen hundred quarts a day to Philadelphia. By midsummer, breaker boys were riding freight trains into the Catawissa Valley to steal potatoes from farmers' fields and to make off with their meat birds.

With miners gone from the mines and the mules pulled from the ground, a great mischief of rats came climbing out of the earth, up through narrow passageways, erupting out of every driftmouth and shaft opening, streaming into every mine patch, and covering every culm bank. And behind the rats came thousands of cops. Every day for weeks, they arrived on trains from Philadelphia and New York, filling every barracks in every coal camp and colliery yard. And not just to work as Coal and Iron cops. The independent coal companies in Hazleton hatched a plan to transform private police into a kind of permanent posse, one that could use overwhelming force under color of law and patrol beyond the stockades, anywhere and everywhere the miners could be found. They called it the Flying Squadron.

CHAPTER FOUR

THEY CALLED IT THE FLYING SQUADRON

The coal companies filed so many requests for police commissions that the state ran out of application forms. Some of the newly hired cops were company clerks reassigned to guard duty, the rest were hired by labor agents who walked up to men on the street and offered them jobs on the spot. The Philadelphia agencies advertised in the papers for out-of-town watchmen at $2.50 a day, experience running pumps and boilers preferred. We'll put you up in barracks, they said, and give you all you can eat, liquor and tobacco included. By the end of May, twelve hundred newly commissioned Coal and Iron cops were patrolling the collieries *with the same watchfulness maintained over camps in times of war.* At every large coal mine, gangs of carpenters surrounded collieries with rough-sawn lumber stockades topped with barbed wire. They installed electric light plants for powerful searchlights to turn night into day. Inside the stockades they built barracks and commissaries to house and feed guards and replacement workers. Three weeks into the strike, the Philadelphia and Reading Coal and Iron Company had an army of 350 private police standing guard over five thousand scabs. By the middle of summer, thousands more worked at collieries throughout the coalfields, cleaning culm in the washeries or stoking the boilers that ran the pumps that kept the mines free of water.

By June, with nearly five thousand private cops in the coalfields, the mine owners began their usual public relations campaign, trying to sway public opinion to their side by painting the miners as unruly, the union as un-American, and their demands as unreasonable. Our relations with the miners *were very pleasant,* they claimed, but *the advent of unionism* established *a spirit of unrest, discontent, and hostility* among the miners. We admit there's *dissatisfaction amongst the men,* but it's not low wages or dangerous working conditions that causes it. Rather it's the false promises of the radical union organizers, which undermines *individual effort, curbs ambition, and limits their earning capacity.* When we pay higher wages, they show no *desire for work.* They are unmanageable now, and it's because their leaders have created a *spirit of insubordination.* This class of labor *doesn't appreciate or understand our institutions.* The miners can't see this because they're led by unmanly, un-American, and un-Christian union leaders who prevent honest men from working. Combinations of labor threaten all the things our *free American life makes necessary to the happiness and well-being of our people.* This strike will provoke a coal famine and threaten industrial stability everywhere, which shows this union is led by *gross agitators.* Mitchell is the worst of them, they insisted. He talks of conciliation and presents himself and the UMW as conservative, but his true aim is to put the collieries under his control and he won't stop until they *secure control of the government.* Oh, what a surly, undisciplined lot they've become. *They won't listen. A man, or a boy, will stand up and tell you, after giving him an order, I won't do it.* He'll look you in the eye and say, *Johnny Mitchell is my boss.* They don't know their place. The union men freeze out the nonunion men. They heckle and harass him until he quits. *Don't you know you're a scab? What do you want to go on taking another man's place for?*

They complained about the boys who worked in the breakers. What kind of union is it, they asked reporters, that puts boys in charge of their own union locals? The breaker boys hold their own union meetings and come out demanding higher wages, shorter hours, sleigh rides on demand. If they don't get their way, they shut down the breaker. We pay them good wages and offer them night school, but these boys are incorrigible. They see how the union men come and go as they please and work when they want. They learn the same bad habits. The miners think they have the right to control everything. They'll boycott a milkman if he sells milk to a scab. Children walk out of school if a teacher's father or brother takes a miner's job. Priests abandon the pulpit if a scab sits in a Sunday pew. They are not so easy to handle now as they used to be before the strike of 1900. You should hear them. They *use some very mean names against us.* Enough is enough. *To hell with the union.*

These were their familiar tactics, used by the companies in every strike, from the advent of wage labor until the strike of 1902. If a wage cut resulted in walkouts, axe-wielding foremen forced them back to the mines. If walkouts continued, the mine owners blacklisted the union organizers and evicted the union miners. If this provoked marching and picketing, the mine owners flooded the anthracite region with thousands of Coal and Iron Police. If wildcat strikes turned into a general strike, they brought in the detective agencies to infiltrate the union. The 1897 Lattimer massacre, however, marked a turning point. An organized *belligerency and fearlessness* emerged among the eastern European miners. They joined the union in large numbers and demanded that it defend their interests. They refused to cross picket lines and attacked the men who took their jobs. Their violence seemed otherworldly. If a foreman tried to break up their pickets, they beat him until his kidney ruptured. When scabs took their jobs, they chased after them, throwing cobblestones and firing pistols, and when they caught them, they clipped their ears, marking them as scabs, and then pitched them into creeks. They stormed jails and staged jailbreaks when their comrades were arrested.

The discipline, solidarity, and quick violence of the eastern European miners made the otherwise conservative United Mine Workers suddenly unpredictable. Some union locals maintained friendly relations with colliery bosses, even inviting them to the union meetings. Others chased them out with clubs and axes. This unpredictability complicated the recruitment of private police and scabs. At the start of the strike, the Lackawanna sheriff offered five times the miners' wages for private policing work but found no takers. Men once accustomed to making easy money as scabs now saw all the effigies hanging from the telegraph lines and heard all the stories of scabs being clubbed and stoned and thought twice about being a fink. When thousands of firemen and pumpmen joined the strike in mid-June, scores of collieries were forced to shut down their pumps and watch the mines flood with water.

Union leaders, always worried about public opinion, tried to tamp down on this new militancy. They scattered fifteen thousand copies of strike instructions throughout the region, ordering the strikers to stay away from the mines. *Avoid being drawn into quarrels or disputes. Be law abiding. Use intoxicants with extreme moderation and practice strict economy with your money. When you confront the scabs, keep your cool and don't break the law when you solicit them to cease work; avoid mingling in large crowds, and above all, listen to your union leaders and cooperate with us. We've earned the esteem and goodwill of the public, don't squander it.* The strikers, however, had other ideas. They organized enormous parades in every mine patch and town, holding flaming torches above their heads and banging pots and pans together. They raised banners aloft on which they'd written threats in English and Polish: *Scabs must leave town, Death to Scabs.* Most parades included fife and drum corps, buglers, or brass bands. They marched from one scab's house to another, stopping at each to throw rocks and tin cans. They made effigies out of old miners' clothes stuffed with plantain leaves and garden rubbish and hung them in front of every scab's house. They strung banners across bridges emblazoned with the names of every scab in town. A parade of strikers marched in a solemn procession through the streets of Miners' Mill, and when they got to the home of Will Martin, son of the Lattimer killer James Martin, they surrounded it and staged a mock funeral while the band played Handel's "Dead March." Every parade ended at a colliery or washery where hundreds and sometimes even thousands of marchers blocked nonunion workers from entering or leaving. Striking breaker boys on bikes ferried messages back and forth between sentries posted at trolley and train stations and the paraders on the march.

Scabs told tales of vicious beatings. *One of the women came at me with a club,* said a scab named John Frederick, who tried to pass through a parade in early June. *I grabbed her hand, and I was then surrounded by twenty or twenty-five women, and they pelted me like hail stones, and I made a dive to get through past the women. When I got through there, I ran right into the men. One of them tripped me up, and I fell down and I laid there. I got it good.* When a scab or a boss tried it more than once, the miners seized him, blindfolded him, and marched him out of town. When a scab went to work in the morning, he'd find a freshly dug grave in his yard. When he returned at night, he'd find the words *SCAB HOUSE* painted on the side of his shanty. Polish women threatened to break the legs of scabs' wives. We'll knock out your teeth, they'd say. We'll drive a knife through you when you least expect it. We'll blow up your house with dynamite if you're not careful. Strikers set the Hollenback and Stanton colliery stockades on fire, dynamited the steam pipes, stoned the washeries, overran the barricades, and then destroyed the boiler house. When a colliery superintendent and a detachment of guards surrounded a group of strikers, *a squad of marching women armed with long sticks surrounded them.* When the National Guard occupied Shenandoah in September, the discipline of the pickets, who kept watch at every train and trolley station in every town, stunned the general in charge. They stood on every corner and kept track of every troop movement. *I could not move a column of my troops in any direction,* he complained, *or at any time of the day or night, without finding some people on duty. Even the HQ in my stable were well picketed.* The pickets and parades electrified Mother Jones when she visited Hazleton in August. *Each parade makes them stronger,* she marveled. *Each clubbed deputy makes them more feared.*

The Coal and Iron Police couldn't keep up. They found

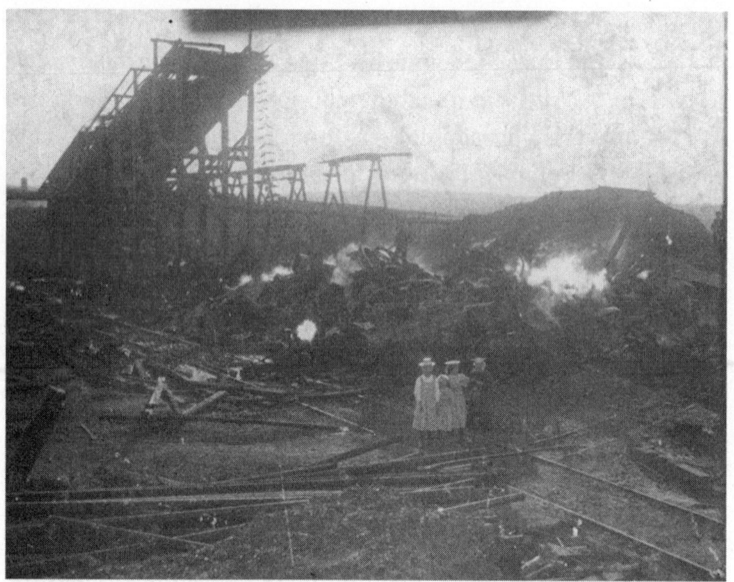

What remained of the Beaver Meadows breaker after it burned down during the 1902 strike. Courtesy: Pennsylvania State Archives.

spiked train tracks, cocked train switches, and bridges on fire. The front porches, pigeon pens, and chicken coops of foremen and scabs began mysteriously blowing up. The Wanamie colliery's enormous culm bank exploded one night, triggering a seventy-ton avalanche that blocked the railroad tracks. Colliery guards found empty dynamite boxes in the woods on the day after an explosion destroyed the Lehigh and Wilkes-Barre's Jersey Annex dam, which shook the town and flooded the mine. Guards at one colliery woke up one night to the sound of explosions and found the ventilation fans destroyed and the pumps that kept the mine clear of water wrecked. Strikers hiding in the woods took pot shots at trains that brought coal out of the washeries. A barrage of stones pelted a Central Railroad of New Jersey train as it traveled through Wanamie, and then again as it passed through Auchincloss. It almost jumped the tracks when it hit a great pile of lumber and old ties stacked on the tracks near Warrior Run. The conductor, taking cover from stones and bullets, missed an open switch at Sugar Notch and drove the train into the back of another at full speed. When dynamite derailed an eighteen-ton Lehigh and Wilkes-Barre lokie steam engine, the cops found a note addressed to the *Scabs and Blacklegs.* Take heed of our warning, the note read, *Ye vile dogs of SATAN.*

When the largest collieries hired more cops to guard their collieries, the crowds grew even larger and more aggressive. When the Lehigh & Wilkes-Barre's Stanton colliery hired more scabs and tried to restart its boilers, a crowd estimated in the thousands attacked the stockades. A line of newly hired cops stood inside the fences and opened fire. All at once, the enormous crowd dropped to the ground as the sound of gunfire echoed through the narrow valley. *I was in a crowd of boys several hundred feet from the colliery,* said twelve-year-old Charlie McCann, who was sitting atop a culm bank watching the attack. *I was only looking on.* A bullet pierced his shoulder and sent him tumbling headlong down the culm bank. Dozens of strikers raced to his aid, while hundreds more turned and attacked the cop who fired the shot, tearing down the stockades to chase after him, and setting fire to the breaker to flush him out. They shoot children now, reported the papers. The Brotherhood of Railroad Firemen announced it would not use nonunion coal to fire their engines. The barbers of North Scranton began refusing to shave the faces of the nonunion men.

Suddenly, the old strikebreaking tactics no longer worked. But only the largest operators were even trying. The independent operators had already begun looking for alternatives. When a Philadelphia detective agency offered its strikebreaking services to L. C. Smith of Coxe Bros. & Co. prior to the start of the strike, Smith had his clerk, E. A. Oberrender, write back and decline the offer. *In past years we have had considerable secret service work done by the Pinkerton Agency*, wrote Oberrender in early March of 1902, but we have no need for your services this year. Smith and Oberrender had learned their lesson during the strike of 1900. They had hired the Pinkertons to place an agent in the jail, but the agent found that the Irish had *the run of the jail and there'd be no way to place a man in there*. They tried instead to send an agent *pretending to be in the area looking for a bar to buy*, but all Smith and Oberrender got from him were invoices for the beer and whiskey he drank at *Rakatzky's, Hoffmans, and Maloney's* saloons. What's the point of hiring the Pinkertons when their agents just use their cover *as an excuse for spending so much time in saloons*?

Smith proposed a new strategy. *We want to hold the power of employing and arming men with roving commissions*, he explained to Coxe Bros. lawyer Simon Wolverton. *We want to employ emergency men* who can operate under color of law, he explained. Instead of hiring private detectives and building armies of temporary strikebreaking cops, Smith wanted to transform the North Lehigh Coal and Iron Police Association from a small, defensive guard unit into a permanent police force. To do it, he needed to find a way for the police to patrol beyond the colliery fences under color of law. *We cannot let it be shown by the enemy*, he explained to Wolverton, *that some cop who arrested some striker or did the shooting that killed a striker didn't do it as a legalized officer of the law.* Wolverton was skeptical. The North Lehigh cops were just *appointees of the Police Association*, he wrote. As private watchmen, they were prohibited from patrolling beyond the property of the coal companies. While the supplement to the original railroad police statute gave the governor the power to commission private watchmen and coal-company guards *with the powers of policemen of the City of Philadelphia*, it required that they be employed by a colliery. The North Lehigh cops, however, worked for the association, not the collieries directly, and therefore could not be commissioned under the statute. *The safest course*, wrote Wolverton, would be to have some squire or constable do the work for you. Hire private detectives to infiltrate the union, compel the sheriffs to hire special deputies. Leave the arrests and prosecutions to the justices of the peace. But Smith persisted. What if we combined all the private police forces of the Lehigh association into one force? Is there some way we could make them *full-fledged officers of the law*? The only way, Wolverton explained, would be if you filed joint commission requests with the governor. The law doesn't provide for joint commissions, he noted, but it doesn't prohibit them either. Have all fifteen independent coal companies that make up the association sign every police commission request. Begin with the chief of the North Lehigh Association, Isaac Eckert. Have every colliery in the association request his commission, not just the North Lehigh Coal and Iron Police Association itself. His commission, and therefore his authority as a cop, would extend to every county where the companies operate. This would transform the North Lehigh Association into a state-recognized, regional police agency with the legal authority to patrol anywhere in Luzerne, Schuylkill, and Carbon counties, which would give each North Lehigh cop an even greater authority than Philadelphia police. They could patrol behind and beyond the colliery stockades, make arrests without a warrant, and use lethal force at their discretion, all under color of law, and anywhere in three counties. Smith forwarded Wolverton's letter to Oberrender. *Throw aside all ordinary work,* he told him, *and take up the question of police business.*

Oberrender spent a week at the courthouse filing police commissions for every cop at all fifteen association-affiliated collieries, and then another week establishing a new police headquarters adjacent to Smith's office at the Coxe Bros. Drifton colliery. The new North Lehigh Association would need to be highly mobile, so Oberrender arranged to have *two trains of cars ready* at all times, *a coach and a caboose at their service night and day, steam always up on two railroads, the Lehigh Valley Railroad and the D.S.&S,* both of which had spurs that terminated at the Drifton colliery. The existing North Lehigh cops would be separated into guard units and distributed among the collieries. Smith then hired Willard Young to create and command a small, heavily armed, strike force that would operate as a special unit within the larger police force. They called it the Flying Squadron, and it would operate as a kind of riot squad, confronting strikers anywhere they were found. Young was uniquely qualified for the job. He sold black powder to every superintendent and foreman at all fifteen association collieries, so he was familiar with the area. And he had extensive military experience, having occupied Puerto Rico during the Spanish-American War as an officer in the so-called Governor's Troop of the Pennsylvania Cavalry. And he was an experienced strikebreaker, having served on the Lattimer posse in 1897 and as a Coal and Iron cop during the 1900 strike. I want you to *get together a force of reliable men,* Smith told him, *and take charge of them.*

For his first lieutenant, Young hired Schuyler Ridgeway, who'd served with him on the Lattimer posse. As his third in command, he hired Ario Pardee Platt, who'd provided the guns for the Lattimer posse and whose perjured testimony at the 1898 trial had led to the acquittal of every cop charged with murder. They arranged to have every Flying Squadron trooper armed with a heavy police truncheon and a large capacity Luger carbine. They divided the squadron into smaller fire teams, equipping each with Winchester pump-action shotguns and Spencer or Winchester repeating rifles. If a colliery superintendent or a North Lehigh guard requested backup, or a snitch had a tip about a parade heading toward a colliery, the Flying Squadron could use one of its dedicated trains to reach *any point in the territory within twenty or twenty-five miles in less than an hour.*

While nearly every city of any size had police on the payroll, nothing like the restructured North Lehigh Association existed anywhere. The larger force would operate as the first official regional police agency in the United States, with the Flying Squadron acting as the first police special weapons and tactical unit. And yet, despite their guns and all their planning, they still underestimated the power of the miners' new resolve. When Smith ordered the Flying Squadron into the field for the first time, Young marched into Hazleton on the first of June without having scouted the city and short a full squadron of troopers. He assumed the miners would be disorganized and undisciplined, like they'd been in every previous strike. What Young didn't know was that the union had been posting sentries at all the courthouses and taking note of which collieries filed police commissions and where those police were being posted, then using that information to organize its pickets and parades.

On the night before the Flying Squadron arrived in Hazleton, Squire Daniel McKelvey took his usual rounds and was surprised to find the streets full of strikers. The miners were waiting for the Flying Squadron on nearly every streetcorner. *The men were all sitting there on the public road. Some were sitting alongside the fires playing cards; others were telling stories. Some were standing up.* McKelvey marveled at the sheer number of pickets, and *what good pickets they were*, he noted. As a boy, he'd worked in the breakers alongside the sons of Polish and Italian mine workers, and he spent that night and much of the next day paying his respects to the miners, warming himself over their barrelfires, and chatting in Polish with the Poles and telling jokes in Italian to the Italians.

Young's plan was to take the troopers on a tour through Hazleton as a show of force, and then spend the night at the Hazleton House Hotel before marching onto Drifton in the morning. But when he saw that he was outnumbered, he requisitioned a wagon at a livery to get his troopers off the street and headed directly for the hotel. As they rode down Hemlock Street, a thousand strikers and their supporters lined the road, yelling insults at them as they passed: Scabs! Dogs! Sons of bitches! They arrived to find the hotel surrounded and the entrance blocked. Thomas Duffy, UMW District 7 president, was waiting for them at the head of the crowd. *Are you not workingmen yourselves? You're taking bread and butter out of the mouths of people who are just trying to get more wages here. How would you like it if your own wages were beaten down?* He offered to pay their fare back to Philadelphia. Ridgeway pointed his carbine at Duffy, which scattered the crowd, allowing the troopers to push their way into the hotel, where they spent a restless night listening to the strikers parading up and down the street, taunting them to sleep.

When Young woke the next morning, he found a few of his troopers AWOL. He assembled the rest and marched to Drifton, where a furious Smith was waiting for him. *You're not doing what you're supposed to do,* he told Young. Your job is to confront strikers and make arrests, not hide in hotels. Incite a riot if you need an excuse to pull your weapons. The crowd was enormous, Young explained, *and I only had limited time* to form the unit—*I think 4 or 5 days. I only had six of the right kind of men.* Smith ordered Oberrender to have Duffy arrested, but the Hazleton constables refused. It's not my job *to get the poor miner to buckle on the shackles of serfdom*, responded McKelvey, *and return again under the lash of your cold blooded and sordid clients. The only people engaged in attempted breaches of the peace are the armed thugs who are masquerading under the guise of law.*

Smith ordered Young to reassign all Flying Squadron troopers who lacked strikebreaking or military experience and to fire those he suspected of holding union sympathies. Smith then created two new units to work alongside the Flying Squadron. He first hired the notorious strikebreaker Bartholomew Flynn, a former Chicago police detective well known to the miners for his role in sending four innocent men to their deaths in what became known as the Chicago Haymarket affair. When Flynn was fired from the Chicago Police Department for manufacturing evidence in a different case, he turned to strikebreaking and Smith put him in charge of a small advance scout unit that would provide surveillance to the Flying Squadron. Smith then appointed Oberrender to take charge of what he called the Secret Service Department, an in-house intelligence and infiltration unit that would do the work the Pinkerton Detective Agency once did. Oberrender's job would be to gather tips and lead undercover investigations. He found his snitches among the Coal and Iron cops, constables, squires, postmasters, bank clerks, scabs, breaker bosses, grocers, street peddlers, saloon keepers, and widows. He hired local newspaper reporters as labor spies because they didn't look suspicious when they showed up in town asking questions. He hired Billy Evans of the *Hazleton Sentinel,* who's tactic was to hire strikers for a few dollars to pass out railroad passes and put up posters advertising upcoming fairs and festivals. He'd tell the man that the newspapers needed it publicized, and then he'd spend a few days traveling with the man from town to town, probing him with questions and meeting all his friends and comrades. They'd stop in saloons in every town, and Evans would buy whiskey, beer, and good cigars for anyone willing to talk. Oberrender also hired a reporter named John James, who was less reliable but useful for his willingness to perjure himself for a fee.

There was nothing particularly innovative about any of the specific strategies that Smith brought together in the reconstituted North Lehigh Association. The police were like a tree with gnarled branches, all of which bore familiar fruit. The police mandate to impose order was already enshrined in law. The use of heavily armed strikebreakers was an existing strategy. Labor spies and snitches had long worked for the coal companies. And while the Coal and Iron Police couldn't patrol from town to town under color of law, sheriffs deputies and posses could. The coal companies used some combination of all of these tactics in every strike. But the reconstituted North Lehigh Association turned out to be less like a bushel of bad apples harvested from a rotten tree, and more like a new branch of police grafted onto an old tree that bore new and unexpected fruit.

Law delegates to police the authority to impose order. While law limits police enforcement to practices consistent with general legal principles, it also extends to individual police officers the discretion to determine what constitutes an emergency and who constitutes a threat. Over the course of the next four months, the North Lehigh Coal and Iron Police Association offered proof of concept for a new and novel variety of the police. The cops of the North Lehigh Association declared every striking miner a potential threat to law and order and every parade and group of pickets a state of emergency. As a newly formed permanent police department staffed by experienced military officers operating under color of law with a jurisdiction extending across and beyond existing political boundaries, the North Lehigh Association claimed the discretion, and now held the legal authority, to impose order however its officers saw fit, wherever they patrolled, and for however long they determined necessary, and all of it under the protection of a law they applied however they saw fit.

The new strategy debuted in late June, when a crowd of strikers led by a miner named Dan Mulraney began stopping Coxe Bros. & Co. miners from going to work. Among the people Mulraney stopped was a Coxe Bros. & Co. engineer named Albin Wassmer, who worked as one of Oberrender's snitches. Smith ordered Flynn's unit to get the names of the miners who marched with Mulraney and to keep track of their movements. When Flynn uncovered the strikers' plan to march on the Drifton colliery, Smith sent the Flying Squadron into the field after them. I want this crowd *avenged,* ordered Smith.

The next day, as three hundred marching strikers armed with pistols, clubs, and miners' needles crested the hill on a march to the Drifton colliery, they found the Flying Squadron waiting for them, blocking the road. When they were within earshot, Young read the riot act and ordered them to halt. The miner leading the march, Duff Shovlin, raised a hand to stop the marchers. Wait! he yelled to the cops. He turned and told three men standing with him to announce a retreat. When the marching strikers turned, Young ordered the Flying Squadron after them. Instead of retreating with the rest of the marchers, Shovlin and the three miners with him stood their ground and hurled insults at the cops as they came. The Jeddo miner John Waskevicz called them dogs. John Shrader, another Jeddo miner, called them *sons of bitches. They have no more right on the street than we have.* The Upper Lehigh miner William Gelgot, another of the three standing with Shovlin, told one of Young's troopers what he'd do to him if he got him alone in Freeland. Eckert told him to shut his mouth, and when Gelgot refused, Eckert raced forward, grabbed him by the shirt, and wrestled him to the ground. Two other troopers ran forward and dragged Gelgot back to their waiting train, beating him with clubs as they went. Eckert turned toward Waskevicz and lunged at him, but Shovlin pushed him away. *What right do you have to stop these men? You're trash*, said Shovlin to Eckert. He pulled his army and navy gun from its holster and pointed it at Eckert. Is this worth it to you? Shovlin yelled. Before the strike you men *worked for ninety cents a day, and now you're getting two and half a day, but after this thing is over Coxe Bros. & Co. will throw you out*, he said. *If you try to take any of us, I'll shoot one of you*, but Eckert hit him in the face with a billy club before he could finish his sentence, knocking him to the ground. Two troopers wrestled the gun from his hands and dragged him toward the train where Waskevicz, Gelgot, and Shrader were already under arrest for rioting and conspiracy. The Flying Squadron railroaded the four strikers to Weatherly, where they were held without bond for trial.

The success of the new strategy convinced Smith to expand Flying Squadron operations. They spent the month of July confronting crowds of marching miners in city after city—Old Forge, Drifton, Nanticoke, and South Wilkes-Barre. They broke up parades, arrested leaders on trumped-up charges, tying up the union in legal fight after legal fight. Strikers tried to exhaust the Flying Squadron by marching during the day and setting bonfires at night in front of Coxe Bros. and Co. collieries. The Flying Squadron responded by ignoring the marching crowds and instead escorting scabs to and from the collieries under armed guard, which allowed colliery after colliery to restart the boilers and clear the mines of water. Unable to block the scabs from going to work, the strikers declared a boycott of all Sheppton and Oneida scabs, threatening to burn down the stores of any merchants who defied it. But Smith had options now. He ordered the Secret Service Department to find out who was behind the boycott. Oberrender spent months collecting tips, taking affidavits from merchants and scabs, interviewing the mothers and sisters of boycotted scabs fired from teaching jobs. He gathered information from Catholic priests who told him they were too scared to anoint a sick scab or give Last Rites. He recorded the number and location of effigies found hanging from telegraph lines and cataloged the signs that hung from them (e.g., *John Foote, the bloody scab; Albert Catley's Last Chance).*

Prior to the start of the boycott in Sheppton and Oneida, Oberrender had been trying to make a case against UMW District 7 president William Dettery, whom Smith wanted arrested for confronting a coal shoveler named Jerry Derr. According to Derr, who had refused to go out on strike with the union, Dettery had said to him, *don't you think you should come out and stand by us? We'll stand by you. The company doesn't care for you.* But Derr had refused, telling Dettery his loyalties were with his foreman Charles Rohland. *I work at anything Rohland has charge of and anything he tells me to go at I'm going to do.* The next day, Derr found large, printed posters nailed to every tree in Nuremburg and Derringer, big signs with huge letters no one could miss.

JERRY DERR
Shun him! Despise him!
A SCAB is a man without soul or principle.

Derr ripped a sign off a tree and took it to Rohland, who showed it to Smith, who ordered Oberrender to find out who printed the posters, who posted them, *and anything else we can use legally.* Tips concerning the strike activities of union officers had the highest priority. The arrest of a union official on a conspiracy charge was the quickest route to an injunction against the union, which nearly always ended a strike. The union would be barred by law from marching and posting pickets. Derr claimed Dettery confessed to making and hanging the posters. I confronted Dettery about the posters, he told Oberrender. I told him I'd take it out of any man who tried to have me boycotted. *Then take it out of me,* he said Dettery told him.

After taking Derr's affidavit, Oberrender went to Sheppton to look for the man Derr claimed had proof of Dettery's role in arranging the boycott, which was the same day that Mulraney's crowd stopped Wassmer from going to work. Smith ordered Oberrender to suspend the Derr case for now and return to Drifton. We'll get Dettery later, he told him. For now work up an arrest warrant against Mulraney. Oberrender spent the next two days taking sworn statements from Flynn, Eckert, and the other cops in Flynn's unit, all of whom told the same story—big crowd, lots of insults, riotous behavior. All agreed it was Mulraney who stopped Wassmer, who happened to be one of Oberrender's most reliable snitches. It had been Wassmer's reports on Mulraney that Flynn has used when first scouting his crowds. Wassmer had first argued with the pickets on June 6, demanding they let him pass. They laughed at him and called him a scab. *We are the right,* they told him, *and we are the law now.* Day after day, he filed reports about the crowd. On June 7: *Came to the same crossing and met the same refusal.* Same thing on June 8: *Tried to go through but without success.* His report on June 10: *I was rejected.* He nearly snuck through the blockade on June 11, when he *tried to make the electric car but was not successful.* Flynn told Oberrender that some of the cops in his unit had witnessed Mulraney attack Wassmer, but when Oberrender took their affidavits, he found that none of them had actually seen anything. Even Wassmer was vague when he talked to Oberrender. *I met a mob of about 300 people,* he told Oberrender. *All strangers to me except one who I can identify but whose name at this time I don't know.*

Oberrender interviewed Flying Squadron troopers next. Young told him he'd seen a railway fireman stopped by the crowd the same day as Wassmer. Oberrender tracked the man down in Drifton and took his affidavit. *A man named Mulraney caught Wassmer by the throat, he told Oberrender, and the crowd threw him to the ground beating him with clubs and insisted on his returning to his house which he refused to do, they then crowded and pushed him up the street.* Oberrender showed the fireman's affidavit to Flynn, but all Flynn would testify to was how heroically he'd *preserved the peace and good order* despite all the slurs thrown at him. The rest of Flynn's unit could only say how difficult the job was what with all those people calling us *thugs.* Oberrender knew the lawyers wouldn't file an arrest warrant against Mulraney until he could corroborate the fireman's story. He turned to John James, finding him drinking at the Centre Hotel bar in Freeland. James said he couldn't remember if he'd seen anything, but a promise of regular work might jog his memory. I'd like to help you, but you have *to deserve it* first, Oberrender told him. Yes, I remember now, James said. *I saw Wassmer walking down Centre Street.* Suddenly, *hands were laid upon him by a man named Daniel Mulraney.* Wassmer protested but Mulraney pushed, jostled, and jeered him past *Boyles saloon where Wassmer again tried to explain to them his position when he was struck over the head with clubs by parties in the mob.* Oberrender hired James to track down all the men stopped by the crowd, explaining to him that he needed at least one other witness willing to swear that Mulraney attacked Wassmer.

Oberrender then showed James's affidavit to Wassmer, hoping the snitch would claim it as his own, or at least understand what was needed from him. But all this did was confuse the snitch, who launched into a bizarre story about being assaulted but somehow not being a witness to his own assault. *A sailor named Franch who works at No. 1 Drifton was present when I was assaulted. A Hungarian called the Dude who does his drinking at John Hudock's was the first man to push me back when I raised my hand, and Mulraney caught me at the neck. Deach, from Upper Lehigh, hit me with a club. This was told to me by my men who said that young Rugan said he saw it. I can't get any more evidence now, must go at it diplomatic. Can't rush in.* The sailor might not be a good witness though. He *denies being there when I was struck.*

By mid-July, more than a month after the alleged attack, Oberrender had a victim who didn't know how to act like one, and conflicting accounts from all the cops. He told Smith he'd hit a dead end, but Smith ordered him instead to *push the matter faster.* Oberrender showed up at James's house uninvited. *I'm very much disappointed in your work,* Oberrender told him. You made certain promises *but haven't delivered. We haven't received a single report.* James protested. I've been doing my best, I promise. I've been interviewing a great many people in Freeland, but I haven't been able to learn much of anything on the Wassmer case. *I didn't want to send you a report about nothing,* he said, pulling out his notebook, flipping through it, reading aloud the names of all the men he claimed he'd interviewed. I found only one who *claimed to be an eyewitness to the attack on Wassmer. Name is John Boyd. The problem is he didn't see who struck Wassmer, though he told me he saw the entire crowd rush upon him, including Mulraney.*

Oberrender decided to give up on James. He told him to drop the investigation and spend his time instead getting *the feeling of the people about Freeland on the relief they were getting from the United Mine Workers.* He returned to Drifton and wrote up a backdated description of Mulraney's alleged attack on Wassmer, corroborating the fireman's affidavit, inventing a plausible scenario. He called the crowd *a riot, a mob armed with clubs.* They attacked Albin Wassmer. He *was sworn at, called vile names, assaulted, knocked down, kicked, beaten into insensibility, head and face cut, body bruised—laid off from work for days.* He then gave the embellished summary, along with the perjured affidavits, to the Pottsville lawyers, who used them to swear out a warrant against Dan Mulraney, who was arrested and held *under bond for trial.* Oberrender didn't care that

Mulraney would later be acquitted. His job was to impose order, not enforce the law.

With the Mulraney case closed, Oberrender turned his attention to the case of John Harvilla, who'd gone out on strike with the rest of the miners but had crossed the picket line when his children started *crying for bread. I had nothing to eat, and I asked for help, and the union said you have a cow, you can kill and eat it.* In late August, after returning from work one night, a man calling him a scab pounded on his door and demanded that he come out. Harvilla peeked out the window and saw other men standing in the street. Frightened, he spent the night hiding in a corner of the front room holding a hatchet. In the morning, when the street was clear, he ran to work and told his foreman, who told Smith, who put Oberrender on the case. *Determine whether we have a case*, he told him. *We want to fight it if we can.* Oberrender traveled to Beaver Meadow by buckboard and interviewed Harvilla. I'd been walking home that night, said the scab, *and shortly after I reached home a Jew from Hazleton was in the road near my house selling apples and wanted to sell me some, but a man named Mike Winell came along there and said to the Jew: Don't sell apples to the scab.* Harvilla ran into the house. *I didn't go out then for the apples—I was afraid.* I figured it was over, but then Winell came up to my door *with a stone in one hand and a stick like a policeman's club in the other hand and called me a son-of-a-bitch, God-damn-scab, and everything bad, and said if I don't catch you tonight, I will get you some other time. He also threatened my wife.* Then *a big crowd gathered in the road and about my house during this trouble, and they were there about an hour when Mike Winell went home, then Mike Salako, another boarder from the same house, came to my house and hollered for other people to hold me that he wanted to kill me and to hit me with a stone. I stayed in the house, back of the door, with an axe and hatchet, I asked my wife what I should do, she told me to keep as quiet as I could, after while Salako went away*. The next night was quiet, which was a relief because I was getting nervous, but then *a lot of boys and some men with them came to my place and hung an effigy along the public road on the telegraph pole, just across the road from my house.*

Oberrender later checked with the mine foremen and they all confirmed Harvilla's story about the effigy, telling Oberrender that they'd sent a man to pull it down. The crowd returned, Harvilla continued. They surrounded my house and called me vile names. I ran upstairs and peeked out a window, but when I drew the window blind to take a peek, a shotgun blast struck me in the face. Harvilla's wife rushed him to the miners' hospital outside Hazleton where doctors removed what was left of his right eye. And then they showed up again, a week later, pounding on the door and trying to climb through a window. They kept hollering for me to come out. *Leave me alone. I've had enough trouble in losing my eye. And the people said, we won't go off before we pull your other eye out.*

Smith wanted warrants filed against Winell and Salako, but Oberrender couldn't find a corroborating witness, and worse still, Harvilla kept changing his story. He said he got shot peering out the window. Then he said he got shot pulling down the effigy. *It was about seven o'clock in the evening.* I was standing close to the telegraph post swinging a long stick at the effigy like it was a piñata. *I don't know who done it for it was pretty dark, but they shot at me out of a gun.* The blast knocked me to the ground and took out my eye. Oberrender considered closing the case, but then changed his mind when he got a tip from a North Lehigh cop who said his son had overhead the Gordon boy bragging about how his father had been the one who shot Harvilla's eye out. Oberrender gave the case to Evans, who went to Beaver Meadow pretending to be a reporter writing a story about the shooting. He found John Gordon giving out relief orders to striking miners. He introduced himself and when Gordon mentioned having to go to the post office, he offered to give him a ride, making sure to pass Harvilla's house on the way. *See there,* Gordon said, pointing to the house, *damn scab got shot right there.* Evans pretended to be surprised. *Is that right? Were you the one who did it?* No, Gordon said. *Yesterday Mrs. Harvilla was at the spring for water. She met my mother-in-law there and told her that it was me who shot her man. People are saying it's me. I got a shotgun and maybe people think it was me,* he said, smiling. *But I got plenty witnesses to prove me not near Harvilla's house when he was shot.*

Evans thought Gordon was being coy, so he stopped at a saloon and bought Gordon a drink. *What's new in the Meadows?* he asked when their drinks arrived. *Nothing's happened here since the scab got shot,* said Gordon. The talk of Harvilla brought more miners to the conversation. *I'm the one they're blaming for it,* Gordon told the crowd. Don't worry, a delivery driver from Coleraine told him. *They can't fasten that on you. I seen you down here at the time the first shots were fired out of the revolver. Me mother and those seven other women who were sitting on the porch at the time can testify as to your being down here when the first shots were fired.* Gordon said that was good to know, and then he launched into a long speech about the shooting and all the rumors, saying, *I ain't the least bit alarmed about the charges made against me.* Evans was getting impatient, so he *put plenty of beer into the whole crowd to keep everyone talking,* but never once did Gordon *leave anything drop that could be picked up to form a link.* Even later, when Gordon *was feeling his beer pretty well,* and Evans *put him through a course of sharp questioning* on the trip back to Beaver Meadow, the only thing Gordon would say was that he was glad to have made a new friend in Evans and wanted his address so he could bring him *several rabbits when hunting season opened.* Evans filed a report recommending that Oberrender close the case. *If Gordon was the guilty man he has plenty of witnesses to prove his whereabouts.* When the lawyers wouldn't file an arrest warrant based on Harvilla's affidavit, Oberrender arranged to have Gordon, Winell, and Salako blacklisted and evicted when the strike ended.

Evans's failure to get an affidavit in the Harvilla case gave Oberrender doubts about him. He was slow, expensive, and hard to reach, like the way the Pinkertons used to work. He was prone to longwinded reports unrelated to cases assigned him. He'd say he'd gotten some young miner drunk and got him to admit to being involved in some plot to dynamite some scab's house, but *don't have him arrested yet. He'll come in handy to me later.* Some of his reports were just updates about how promising some mark might be in the future. I have plans to *get him drunk for the next three days and nights, and I think things will come my way o.k.*, but then weeks would pass, and nothing would come of it. Or he'd promise he was *in it proper for a scheme and satisfied he had the right mark. I'll land information galore through him*, but then all they'd get were requests for more expense money. He always needed more carfare, more money for drinks and cigars, more money for dinners in Hazleton with union officials. In July he said he'd *gleaned considerable information on the boycotting case*, but then said *he had to go mighty slow on the case proper.* Can't deliver anything yet, he said. In due time, he promised. When Oberrender reminded him that the purpose of the Secret Service Department was tying up of the union in constant legal cases, Evans lectured him on union infiltration. *You have to understand, there's no easy road to travel to get the information you want. The fellows down there are on their guard. I have to go slow and work through every tip. This work takes weeks, not days. You're the boss in the case and I'll abide by your decision, but my targets tell me this region doesn't know what trouble is yet. Things are about to get lively, and a movement is on to do some violence.*

Smith decided to fire him, but then Evans reported that he'd infiltrated the Sheppton union local and got himself a copy of the meeting minutes. It came with a roster of every man who attended the boycott meetings and every man assigned to the boycott committee, including Dettery, Evans reported. My mark tells me he was the one who ordered the boycotts. Smith told Oberrender to pay Evans *whatever money he wants*, and to make it clear to him we might need him to *do something desperate*. Dettery had already dodged three arrest warrants. This one had to stick.

According to Evans, the boycott had started in early June, when committees of striking miners started visiting Sheppton and Oneida merchants and leaving behind lists of the men to be boycotted. *You are hereby asked by the U.M.W. of A. that you discontinue selling goods of any kind, even a cigar or shave any of the persons whose names are written on this list.* A few protested, explaining that they'd lose their license if they boycotted the scabs. In those cases, the union allowed them to sell to the scabs but only at higher rates. If a scab tried to buy a shirt, the merchant had to double the price. If a scab ordered a beer in a saloon, the barkeep could charge the regular price but could only serve it half full. The boycott applied to scabs and everyone they were related to. *My family cannot go anywhere over there in any store*, complained a scab named Thomas McNamara. *The little children cannot get a fire cracker on the Fourth of July.*

All they cared about was Dettery, but the only name that appeared on the Oneida boycott notice was John Hudock's, a saloonkeeper and president of the UMW local in Sheppton. When Oberrender examined the meeting minutes, however, he saw Will Hermany's name, a miner who'd gone out on strike but had later crossed the picket line. If Dettery ordered the boycotts, Hermany would know it. Oberrender wrote up an affidavit accusing Dettery and brought it to Hermany's house. Either sign this affidavit or lose your job. Hermany admitted that he'd attended *some of the United Mine Workers' meetings* and he confessed to Oberrender that he'd *heard some action taken on the unfair list*. What about Dettery? Oberrender asked. Yes,

Hermany said, he'd heard that Dettery was the one who ordered Hudock and two other strikers to write out the boycott notices.

Oberrender took Hermany's affidavit to the Pottsville lawyers, but they wanted more evidence before they would file another warrant against Dettery. Oberrender wrote up a second affidavit based on both Evans's report and Hermany's story and brought it to the house of a miner named Frank Kahley, whose name also appeared on Evans's list. I know you were at the meeting where Dettery ordered the boycott of the scabs, he told him, placing the affidavit in front of him. Sign this and keep your job when the strike ends or go to jail with Hudock and Dettery. Oberrender sat back and watched as a panicked Kahley argued with his wife. You wouldn't have got yourself in this mess, she told him, *if you'd have listened to me. But I was compelled to join* the boycott, he protested. What could I have done? *I'll never join a thing of this kind again*, he told Oberrender. Good, said Oberrender. Now sign the affidavit. Kahley, who couldn't read, listened as his wife read the affidavit aloud to him. *I attended the meeting of the Sheppton Local of the United Mine Workers at Reclas Hall. William Dettery ordered the Relief Committee to call on all business men in Sheppton and request them to refuse to sell any goods or do any work for the people who were working at or about the mines. This man Wm. Dettery is also said to be a member of the National Board of the United Mine Workers. Wm. Dettery said in his speech, if you know of anybody working about the mines, catch them and give them a good thumping.* When she finished, she handed it to Kahley, who signed with an *X*. Hudock was convicted of conspiracy and jailed. Dettery was acquitted of the charges, but only after spending the last month of the strike behind bars.

Oberrender kept a detailed diary of the strike that included a careful list of all the outrages and illegal acts that he claimed to have uncovered during the course of the strike. It included the names of strikers accused of intercepting men going to work and the names of strikers suspected of stoning the houses of scabs. It included short summaries of various investigations: the Oneida scab who was *waylaid by masked men* on his way to work; the scab expelled from the Hungarian Greek Society; the father and son who crossed the picket line in September and got thumped by men armed with beer bottles in October; *the Lithuanian priest* who found a threatening note slipped under his door telling him his *life was in jeopardy* unless he stopped *inducing his flock to return to work*; the black powder and fuses stolen from the Beaver Meadow Powder House; the sabotaged drainage tunnel in Beaver Meadow; and the long list of fences torn down and train tracks spiked or soaped. In mid-October, Smith asked Oberrender to take his list of miners who'd been investigated by the Secret Service Department and convert it into a blacklist, so he'd know who to fire when the strike ended. But there would be no use for a blacklist if the companies couldn't defeat the strikers and force the miners back to work. The North Lehigh Association had proved its worth, but it wasn't coalfield wide. To win the strike, they'd need a version of police with an unlimited jurisdiction, like an occupation.

CHAPTER FIVE

THE OCCUPATION OF SHENANDOAH

Shenandoah, stronghold of the Molly Maguires, *shut in by high hills* and drained by coal of *color or beauty.* A town of steep streets carved from fields of tangled laurels and scrub oak on the undulating land southwest of Hazleton, pockmarked by cave-ins and culm banks, torn open by shafts and strippings, crisscrossed by three railway lines; its high ground a culm heap, its lowest point a flooded moonscape, the hundred-feet thick seam of coal known as the mammoth vein buried below it, a curse to everything above. A dozen mine shafts and slopes dropped from the surface and pierced the mammoth at its thickest point, entryway to a vast underground catacomb of manways, muleways, and gangways, the workplaces of the Irish miners and later the Poles and Lithuanians, who lived in shanty settlements that lay scattered like debris fields along the road to Gliberton. A crowded town of narrow streets where police killed or maimed Poles and Lithuanians at a rate greater than in any other borough, where more of its underground miners died of rockfalls than in any other place, and where more of its children died of starvation than any other cause.

The presence of the foreign element drew reporters to Shenandoah who told sensational tales of riotous, lawless hordes of *polinky*-drinking Polanders and coarse and unkind *Huns* who lived in hovels, paid no taxes, ate rough food, and terrorized honest American businessmen and merchants. When they gathered for a wedding, the papers warned of drunken mobs roaming the streets. When miners refused a wage cut or walked off the job, the papers blamed the immigrants. The start of every military occupation began with these stories of brewing emergencies. First the short, embellished brevities in local papers describing various outrages. Then the stories of the angry mobs. If Poles celebrated a christening in the Greek Orthodox Church or a union local held a meeting, reporters told of threatening crowds of murderous Huns. If a constable shot a striking miner, the papers called it a riot and blamed the dead man for lacking manliness. If a drunk conductor derailed a train, the papers screamed of a return of Molly Maguirism and blamed the Slavs for spiking the tracks. At some point a citizen's alliance would declare itself formed and the papers would publish its petitions

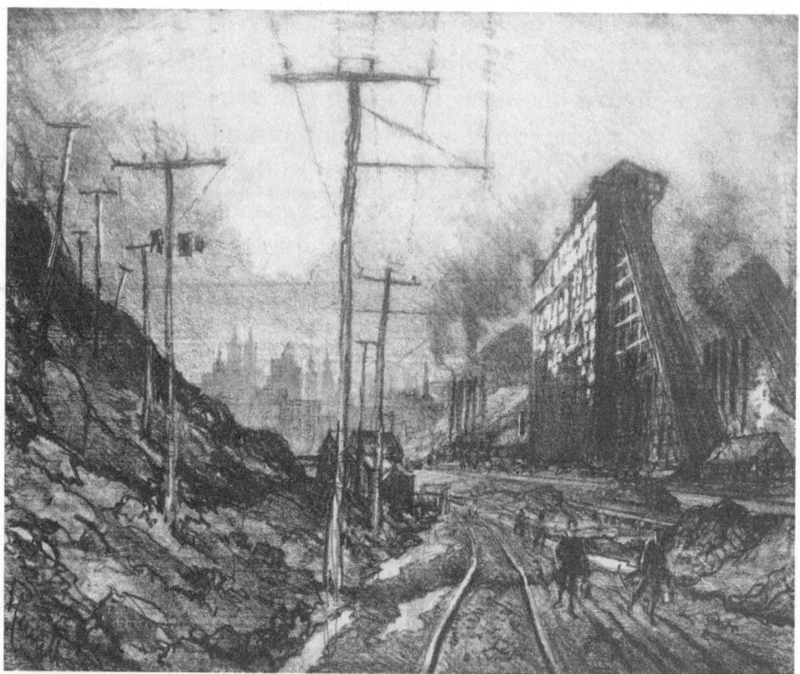

A 1911 Joseph Pennell sketch of the view coming into Shenandoah from Mahanoy City. Courtesy: Library of Congress.

and lists of names of leading businessmen demanding protection. A drumbeat of headlines would follow: *No Police Protection; Beaten Near Mahanoy City; Another Drunken Scrap*. The coal operators would demand protection. Train cars full of strange men would appear. More headlines: *Strikers Arrested; Shot at Girardville; Charged with Riot*. Then a spark—a shooting affray, a shocking murder, an outrage relentlessly reported, telegrams to the governor by prominent citizens—and the Pennsylvania National Guard would march in and declare an occupation. An infantry company in Shenandoah, the cavalry in Mahanoy City, a brigade encampment near Scranton. White canvas tents would be pitched in orderly rows in fairgrounds, ballfields, and racetracks. Headlines would celebrate their arrival: *Military Rule Assures Peace*. A week or maybe a month would pass, and then martial law would be declared, and the entire Pennsylvania National Guard would be called out. Train depots would double as arms depots. Field artillery would be dragged from town to town. Armed troops would march in parades through small towns. Crowds would be called riots, and all riots would be quelled. The solidarity of the miners would fracture. Headlines would predict an end to the strike: *Operators Still Firm; Rioters Routed; Strike Breakers Leave*. The end would come with wage cuts, blacklists, and evictions. Celebratory headlines would fill the papers. *J. P. Morgan Can Settle It; J. P. Morgan in Washington; Miners' Chief in Washington; Rush Coal to Market; Coal has Right of Way*. Starving miners would return to the mines. The union would be crushed. The National Guard would leave.

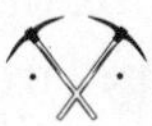

At the end of July, the Philadelphia and Reading Coal and Iron Co. sent two machinists to Shenandoah to fix a broken pump at the West Shenandoah colliery. Deputy Sheriff Thomas Beddall waited at the train station to escort them. When they stepped

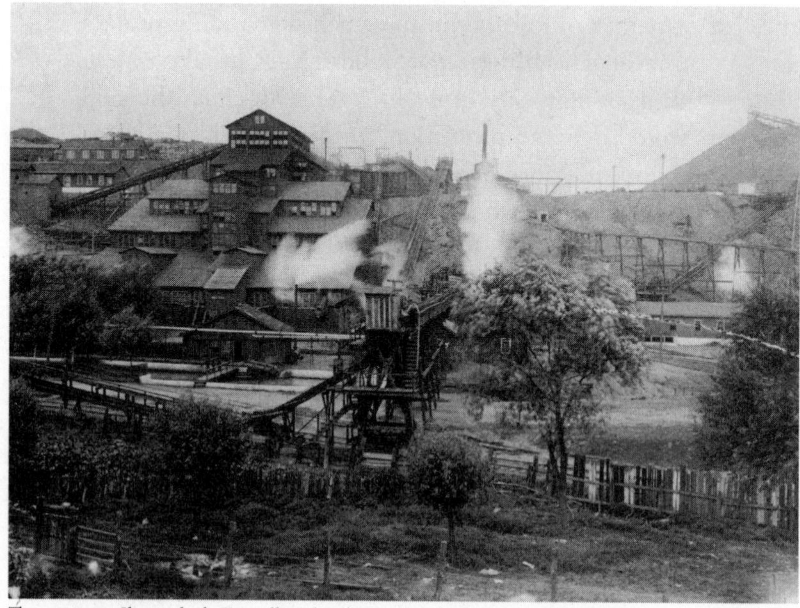

The enormous Shenandoah City colliery breaker surrounded by a mountain of culm.
Courtesy: Indiana University of Pennsylvania Special Collections and University Archive.

off the platform, a crowd appeared demanding to know who they were and where they were headed. Beddall refused to answer and instead pulled his pistol. Get back, he yelled, pulling a copy of the riot act from his pocket. Someone tore it from his hand, and he fired into the crowd, saying later that a woman holding a hatchet gave him no choice. The shooting set off a panic of street fighting. Constables with their guns drawn raced into the crowd. A Lithuanian striker pulled his own gun and fired back. Why did you shoot at the constable? What? Isn't my life *as sweet* as his? In the melee, the first machinist was thrown to the ground and his hat ripped from his head. All around him people were screaming and running. Some said from a man in a second-story window *strafing them with rifle fire.* The second machinist was seen running from a man with an axe. The first machinist fought his way to his feet and scrambled after the second machinist. Beddall, firing at the crowd as he ran, caught up to them as they reached the train depot. They barricaded the door and hid in a baggage room with a wooden-legged man who'd stumbled in after them. By the sound of the rocks hitting the depot, they estimated a crowd in the thousands. They made their escape by leaping into a waiting locomotive from a window in the women's bathroom.

When the crowd dispersed, Joseph Beddall, cousin of the deputy sheriff, was found shot and bleeding in the street. Some blamed the political parties for giving out free beer at their get-out-the-vote parties. He'd been trampled in a panicked, drunken rampage, they said. The coal operators blamed the strikers. In one version of their story, Beddall had been dragged from a saloon by a wooden-legged striker who beat him to death in the street with a four-foot pole. In the version the police told, a Lithuanian butcher and strike supporter named Joseph Paliewicz beat the wooden-legged man, who some say was a scab, before turning the pole on Beddall, a hardware merchant and nephew of Sheriff Rowland Beddall. In a third version, a one-armed saloonkeeper known as Uncle Dan beat the wooden-legged man with a twelve-foot pole and then, in the middle of a riotous crowd, broke the pole into three pieces and used the biggest piece to bludgeon Beddall to death. Some said it was a brick, others swore it was a clothes prop. Either way, most didn't believe Uncle Dan could have done it. Seems like more people would have remembered the sight of a one-armed man beating another man to death in the street.

The miners had their own story. It was the deputy sheriff firing into the crowd and then fleeing on foot that sparked the riot. In the chaos that followed, a scab timberman named Stiney Korkosky, who worked at Lanigan's colliery, beat Joseph Beddall to death with a stick. Korkosky denied it but did himself no favors by constantly changing his story. He claimed at first that Paliewicz killed Beddall with a stick or maybe a billy club but said he couldn't remember which for sure. He also said

Beddall didn't mean to fire into the crowd, it was the beating the miners gave him that *caused the gun to explode*. No one believed him. Saloonkeepers at Tabor's and Nowiski's overheard him bragging about how he'd been paid fifty dollars for *swearing against Paliewicz*. Whenever anyone asked Korkosky about it, his face would blush red. *What makes your face so red, Korkosky?* Are you lying? No, he'd say, *it's the beer I drank an hour ago*. At Paliewicz's trial, the prosecutors admitted that they paid Korkosky, but County Detective Creary said it was just a witness fee and nothing should be read into it. Later it turned out the prosecution paid all the witnesses and even gave them free railroad passes, which clinched it as a fix for most. In November, when Paliewicz was acquitted of all charges, the courtroom erupted in cheering that ended only when the tipstaves waded into the gallery and arrested a breaker boy for cheering too loudly.

Beddall wasn't the only man shot that night. Two striking miners bled to death from gunshot wounds. A half-dozen others, either shot, beaten, or both, walked in the dark to the hospital in Ashland, where doctors dug eighteen bullets from their bodies. When they were released, the sheriff had them arrested for rioting. Beddall was taken to the miners' hospital on the night of his beating, which was the same night the governor called in the National Guard. Beddall was still alive when Brigadier General, and Lieutenant Governor, John P. S. Gobin rode into Shenandoah with two regiments of twelve companies, a cavalry unit, and a battery of field artillery. Beddall died of his injuries the next day, the same day Gobin declared martial law. Dozens of out-of-town reporters followed Gobin into Shenandoah. *The backbone of the strike is now broken*, they wrote, *it will only be a short time until there will be a general resumption of mining.*

Gobin commandeered the Reading Company train depot to store the occupation's weapons and ammunition. For his

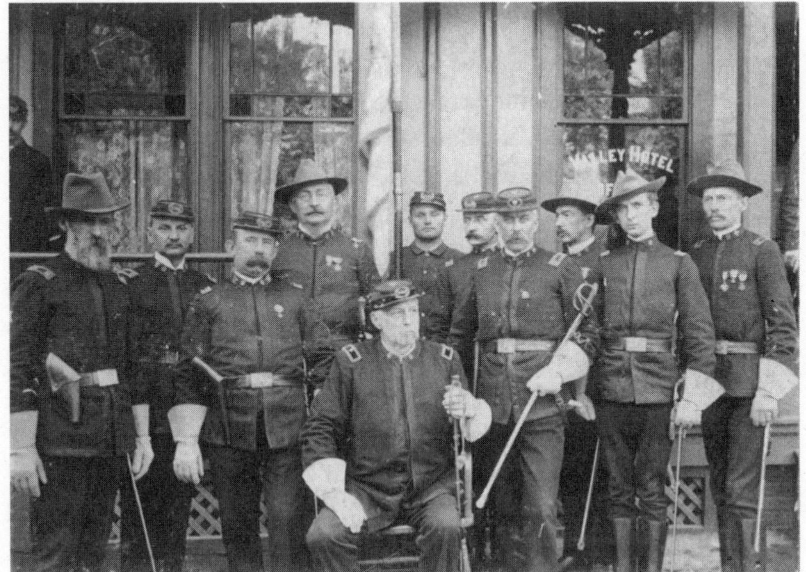

General John P. S. Gobin (seated) and his staff in front of the Valley Hotel in Hazleton during the strike. Courtesy: Pennsylvania State Archives.

headquarters, he took the Ferguson Hotel, where most of the colliery foremen lived. He placed his signal corps on the roof in case the strikers cut the phone lines. Western Union sent a second operator to handle the heavy rush expected at the telegraph office. On the day he arrived, Gobin called the Burgess, but the mayor said he was sick and couldn't meet the general. He called the chief of police, but the chief was in the hospital along with his constables. Gobin sent a provost guard into Shenandoah to clear the streets. *They must depend on me to keep order,* he thought.

Gobin was sixty-five years old with a face and head of snow-white hair that made him look much older. He walked with a cane, hunched when he sat, and squinted when he read. He was born in Sunbury, on the flat ground south of the Susquehanna River's North Branch, where the Six Nations had once come to trade before the settlers arrived. The original settlement was short-lived. Native fighters burned it to the ground in the mid-1700s, but Gobin's great-grandfather claimed *Tomahawk rights* to the land, raised a militia, and resettled the village by force. Gobin studied printing and law until the Civil War interrupted his plans. He fought with the Pennsylvania Volunteers at the battle of Falling Waters, led troops against Mosby's guerrillas at Summit Point, marched through Georgia with Sheridan, served as judge advocate general for the Department of the South, learned the art of military occupation in Key West and Savannah. After the war, he settled near Harrisburg, where he organized returning soldiers into a local militia unit called the Coleman Guards, the first infantry unit of the Swatara Rifles, which later became one of the elite fighting units of the Pennsylvania National Guard's Third Brigade. He was promoted to colonel of the Eighth Regiment in 1874, then brigadier general in 1885. He established a military reserve at Mt. Gretna where he drilled his militia troops on the tactics of a military occupation. A strikebreaking occupation, he taught his troops, was not to be confused with an occupation that followed war. The purpose was not the physical reconstruction and political transformation of a war-torn land but rather a defense of a faltering order. It should begin as small as possible and expand only as needed, and only where strikers were best organized and most active. It should be considered a strength that strikebreaking soldiers came from the same communities they occupied. Invite the local children to watch the marching drill teams. Make a show of the dress parades each night. Stage free concerts by the regimental band and invite the whole town. Gobin taught his officers to control the roads with constant patrols, to interrupt the pickets with frequent arrests, and to make examples out of a few people. Take a child from the home of a striker. Arrest a sympathizer on trumped-up charges. Measure success by the number of strikers who turned scab. Increase the size and intensity of the campaign until solidarity splintered and the collieries reopened. Use lethal force only in the face of open defiance to military authority. Claim that order had been restored only when starvation had broken the back of the strike, and the miners had been driven back underground.

Gobin lost count of the number of times he'd placed his army against the miners. *Whenever troops have been called out, in every strike in the anthracite region, I've served*, he said. He first occupied Shenandoah in 1874 at the start of the Long Strike, when he hunted the Mollies by horseback and troop train from Mauch Chunk to Mahanoy City. Every subsequent occupation followed the same pattern. Tent encampments, armed guards at the train depots, escorts on the trains that brought the scabs to the collieries, daily foot patrols to ferret out the coal pickers, cavalry troops through the mine patches. When he occupied Hazleton in 1875, he brought field artillery, mounted Gatling guns above mine patches, and dug trenches around collieries. His infantry traded fire with strikers in Jeddo. He marched through western Pennsylvania in 1877 during the great railroad strike. He occupied Drifton after the Lattimer Massacre in 1897, placing his guns on the high ground above the site of the massacre and making his occupation headquarters in the Lehigh Valley Coal Company offices. In 1900, he occupied Shenandoah with six infantry companies and a troop of cavalry.

From past occupations, Gobin knew that Shenandoah's livery stables would boycott his troops, so he used the wagons of a Mahanoy City fire company to haul the regimental tents and supplies up the hill to Columbia Park, the forty-acre racetrack along the trolley line to Mahanoy City where his soldiers erected their tents in the infield dirt. He had the camp surrounded by a stockade and ordered the laurel cleared from beyond the fences. They laid pipe to bring water from town, erected a stable for the horses, and built a telegraph station to connect with Harrisburg. While strikers watched from the high ground above the camp, the soldiers spent their first days practicing cavalry charges and using a culm bank for target practice.

Gobin spent the first week of August standing on the roof of the Ferguson, watching the miners ride the trains into Shenandoah to pick up relief funds. He swore he saw the ghosts of the Molly Maguires among them. *The way they jump on and off the freight trains in defiance of the authorities; the way they ride all over the country from one place to another.* He ordered his troops to pull the free riders from the trains. The reporters, crowding around Gobin on the roof, called it an invasion. The Polanders come to scout the troops, they wrote, before skulking off into the woods to their secret camps where they drill in combat tactics in preparation to attack the soldiers. Gobin sent the cavalry into the woods, but they found no camps.

After the first week of August, as a show of force, he sent small details of soldiers into the mine patches and the free towns. Each morning, with their bayonets fixed to their carbines, soldiers in canvas leggings and droopy hats patrolled the streets of Shenandoah. Some strikers turned their backs on them when they passed. Each afternoon Gobin's cavalry rode out to the outlying districts to patrol the nearly deserted mine patches where the only sound was the constant clicking of the mine pumps and the whistles of the faraway trains. They found bridges charred by dynamite or sawed in half by hand tools. They galloped past farms in the Catawissa Valley where German farmers never looked up. They returned to camp through forests of scrub oak and stunted huckleberry, their *faces blackened with coal dust.* Each evening, from his hotel porch, Gobin inspected the soldiers as they marched in dress parades to a cacophony of barking dogs and children yelling Scab! At night the soldiers, barred from the saloons, sang camp songs around barrelfires while listening to the sound of dynamite and gunfire in the distance. During the day, until the soldiers wised up, polite boys and girls wandered into camp with sad stories of

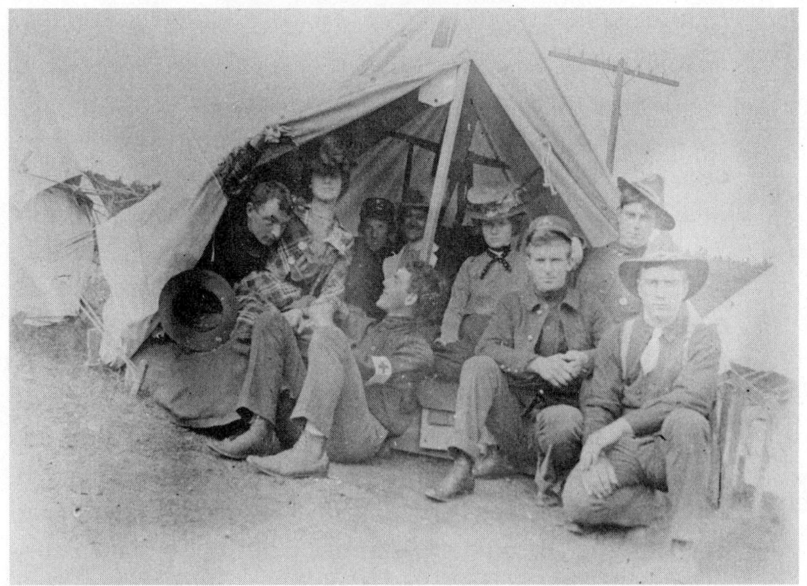

Soldiers posing with Red Cross volunteers in front of a tent in Shendandoah during the 1902 strike. Courtesy: Library of Congress.

drunken fathers and missing mothers, which earned them gifts of bacon and coffee, which they carried home to union fathers and hungry mothers.

One night, during the first week of the occupation, just before midnight, a rock came flying into camp from the laurels, hitting a sentry in the head and knocking him to the ground. He scrambled to his feet and fired blindly into the dark. The regimental commander sent two infantry companies into the bramble, and they chased a stocky Lithuanian man out of the woods just before dawn. He wore a UMW badge on his coat lapel, so they held him in the guard house until Gobin could arrive with an interpreter to interrogate him. What were you doing in the laurel bushes? I was sleeping. Why were you running? Because they were chasing me. Gobin declared him a prolific liar, but what could he do? The constables were all out injured or sick. A guard frisked the man and found a hundred dollars.

Gobin kept the money and let him go. *Maybe it'll keep the man from disturbing us again.*

As soon as the troops arrived, a Shenandoah Citizen's Alliance, which claimed it had the interests of the miners at heart, declared itself formed and demanded more troops. Mitchell called it *a club for capitalists and monopolists.* He traveled to Washington to tell the commissioner of labor, Carroll Wright, that the stories of outrages and unrest in Shenandoah were the exaggerations of the coal operators. All of it was just a pretext to bring the troops and restart the mines, he claimed. *It is the history of past coal strikes that the presence of the militia is always a sure indication of an early resumption of mining.* He told Wright to ignore the operators' claims of poverty. It's all just an accounting trick. The coal companies make plenty of money. You can find the profits of the coal companies in the excessive freight rates of the railroads, which operates like a cartel. Nearly five hundred people in Shenandoah signed a petition demanding the governor remove the troops from Shenandoah, but the governor refused.

Gobin spent his days talking to coal superintendents on the phone, issuing warrants for the arrest of strikers, and threatening to arrest reporters he didn't like. The three phones in his headquarters rang constantly, delivering daily reports of trolley lines cut in Lansford, strikers riding freight trains into the farming districts to steal potatoes, dire warnings of railway tracks soaped where the grade was steepest, and complaints from distant collieries complaining of troop trains stoned and soldiers heckled on patrol (*Scab! Vile dog! Government hobo!*). He talked to superintendents who demanded protection for their scabs. He met with Sheriff Beddall who said his schoolteacher niece Anna, sister to the murdered Joseph Beddall, had been fired from her job and replaced with a strike sympathizer. He sent troops to quell the gangs of strikers harassing scabs in Mahanoy City and Centralia, investigated an outbreak of dynamiting in Frackville, and sent a company to Ashland to extinguish a house fire. The soldiers found the pickets of the strikers everywhere they went. Gobin noticed how different the strike seemed from previous years. The miners were more organized and disciplined than in the past. Support for their cause had broadened to include most of the merchants. In 1900, the arrival of troops in Shenandoah brought a quick end to the strike. But now, in 1902, Gobin fell asleep to the distant sound of dynamite, which seemed to grow closer every night.

Gobin declared the protection of the scabs his primary purpose, but most of those being beaten or killed were striking miners, and the people doing the killing were the Coal and Iron Police, who grew more brazen when the troops arrived. At the end of the occupation's second week, in mid-August, three Nesquehoning cops shot the respected miner and union organizer Patrick Sharpe. When Baird Snyder, the Nesquehoning superintendent, said he was glad Sharpe was killed, the entire population of Nesquehoning attacked the colliery. Snyder's guards couldn't hold the crowd back, and the sheriff begged Gobin for help. *There were hundreds of them. I am powerless. I fear there will be more trouble in the morning.* Gobin marched a battalion of troops into Nesquehoning in the middle of the night—*a secret movement,* he called it—camping them in a public park. When the battalion woke in the morning, it found itself surrounded by an angry, stone-throwing crowd. Whole families, as though at a picnic, came to the park to join the attack. Gobin called a retreat and marched the battalion back to Shenandoah.

Before Gobin could plan a second assault, the coroner released his inquest report. Sharpe had been assassinated, he concluded. It turned out the Shenandoah operators had been planting stories in the papers about Sharpe for months. They first tried to tie him up in the courts by calling him the ringleader behind *all the acts of violence.* Said he was under *bail for five different charges, including highway robbery.* Goes to show that these secret labor organizations are just criminal operations, they told the reporters. When none of the charges stuck, Sharpe grew defiant, and his popularity grew. Baird Snyder sent three cops to rough him up. When they found him, he was going saloon to saloon with the union organizer John Drinkwater, distributing relief funds to immigrant miners and convincing scabs to quit the collieries. Drinkwater recognized the cops as they walked down the street toward them. Good afternoon, Hugh McEmoyle, he said. *Why don't you quit that job you got and come join us?* He figured McEmoyle would smirk, maybe wave him off, but instead McEmoyle called him *a son of a bitch* and knocked him to the ground. Drinkwater tried to get up but William Ronamus, another cop, hit him with an elbow and knocked him back down. *That's when I heard shots fired*, Drinkwater would say later. *I didn't see who shot it. I just looked up and saw Sharpe lying in the street dead.* Thomas Dolan watched the shooting affray from the porch at McCudder's saloon. *They were talking loud*, he said of the cops. *Neither Sharpe nor Drinkwater made any threats.* When McEmoyle hit Drinkwater across the face, Dolan leaped to his feet and made a move to get off the porch, but a third cop, Ezekiel John, pulled a revolver on him. Best get back, he said to Dolan, *or I'll blow your heart out.* While John kept his gun on Dolan, McElmoyle pointed his revolver at Sharpe and shot him in the chest. He then turned and waved his pistol at Dolan and Drinkwater. *I'll give you one too*, he said.

Miners from every union local attended the funeral. More than six thousand marched in the procession that brought Sharpe's body to St. Joseph's church. Five thousand more filled the pews and thronged the streets. *He was shot down like a dog*, said the priest in his eulogy, *a martyr to the miners' cause.* The priest reminded the mourners that Snyder, the superintendent who'd hired the cops and who had celebrated Sharpe's killing, was *a member of the Citizen's Alliance*, and everyone understood what that meant. The operators paid the cops who killed Sharpe, then paid the lawyers who defended McEmoyle and Ronemus, then sent agents and emissaries to cajole and strong-arm witnesses into changing their testimony. Gobin, who wasn't there, called the funeral a riot and described a scene that no one recognized. *Men were assaulted*, he said, *and houses were broken open and furniture thrown in the street.*

Gobin told the governor that he needed more troops to occupy Lansford, Nesquehoning, and Tamaqua—and also that he wasn't happy with the ones he had. There were reports toward the end of August that soldiers were going AWOL. Each payday, the provost guard found soldiers drinking whiskey in saloons with strikers. The coal operators complained that Gobin's troops weren't reliable. We need federal troops, they said. Most of the *State Guard belonged to the miners' union and were in sympathy with its cause.* A Pottsville paper estimated that trade unionists, including striking miners, made up at least half the men in Gobin's command. Gobin said it was true, but it was true in every previous strike too. Their allegiance is to country and flag, he promised, not the miners' union. But then an entire company of troops raised a cheer to John Mitchell when it made its daily march past his headquarters. Gobin admitted to the reporters that he *should have called up the Philadelphia regiments first.* His troops had too close an affinity with the cause of the strikers. They took to shouting scab! when they passed colliery guards. There were reports of fistfights breaking out between soldiers and cops.

The last straw came when Gobin sent two battalions to Tamaqua and Lansford to inspect the trolley track for soap and to see if the lines had been cut. They were jeered when they left Shenandoah and attacked by stones when they pulled into Tamaqua. This can no longer continue, he declared. He issued new orders to his officers. Those who shout Scab! will be arrested. Those who threaten the troops will be shot. When you march, *use your bayonets if at all possible, but place reliable, competent and skilled marksmen on the flanks of your command. They should carry their carbines loaded, and in case of attack by stone or missile, these marksmen shall fire upon their attackers without any further orders. Take note of the saloons where the strikers rendezvous and carefully note such houses and report the names of their owners to headquarters so that application may be made to the Courts for the revocation of their licenses. Keep alert to the disposition of the children and mark those to be taken before the courts for incorrigibility so they can be sent to the House of Refuge.* The governor called it *a wise course to pursue.* No better way to teach these miners *a lesson in good conduct.*

More patrols were ordered. Troops were issued ball cartridges for their carbines, which were more lethal than what they had been using. They began intercepting the cargoes of the beer wagons. Militia officers posted threats on every boardinghouse and hotel. *The harboring of disorderly persons will be met with the closing of the place.* The strikers responded with defiance. Someone threw a rock through a window at the house of the mother of William McElmoyle, one of Sharpe's killers, which knocked over an oil lamp and burned the place to the ground. Dynamite destroyed the Gilberton home of a Draper colliery fireboss. Strikers with straight faces told the press *it must have been a meteor that did it.* Troops on patrol found train tracks dynamited and bridges blown up. A bridge near the Maltby colliery went missing one night. *It must have been cut to pieces and hauled away,* guessed the soldiers. Defiance could not be allowed to take hold, Gobin declared. He added even more patrols and ordered more arrests. His troops began guarding the coal trains that came out of the washeries. In the beginning of September, after the governor ordered out the Second City Troop of Philadelphia, Gobin reinforced it and sent it to Lansford, where it went door-to-door escorting scabs from home to colliery and back.

Gobin predicted the new troops and tactics would end the strike. He had reason to be optimistic. The price of coal spiked to fifteen dollars a prepared ton. Some coal dealers began selling asbestos coal bricks soaked in oil as an alternative. The Hazleton-area mine companies, anticipating the end, sent labor agents into Shenandoah to recruit strikers to work in their collieries as scabs. They were shocked to find no takers. They assumed the miners would be starving and desperate for work, but the bituminous miners of western Pennsylvania donated hundreds of thousands of dollars to a miners' relief fund. A Business Men's Association formed in Shenandoah and Mahanoy City and donated more than a thousand dollars of its own. Doctors began treating strikers and their families free of charge. The UMW opened five stores in Shamokin and started distributing barrels of sugar, flour, and other supplies to any striker who needed it. So much money was donated to the UMW relief fund that the national treasurer said he could take care of the strikers indefinitely. Encouraged, the Shenandoah strikers condemned the dirty tricks of the undercover agents and voted unanimously to remain out of work until the strike was won. The end did seem near, but for once it wasn't the resolve of the miners that was splintering. Typhoid swept through the Shenandoah encampment, killing a soldier in late September. The musicians in the regimental band refused to reenlist. Even Gobin's hometown band refused to serve in the occupation. Troopers began sharing their rations with hungry strikers. Scabs began walking off the job in Shenandoah when the union granted them immunity from attack, but only if they quit immediately. In September, when the schoolchildren of Nesquehoning held their annual back-to-school children's parade, toddlers went from house to house yelling *Scab!* as loud as they could.

At the beginning of October, as the weather turned colder and the prospect of a winter without domestic fuel seemed more and more likely, President Teddy Roosevelt brought Mitchell and the mine owners to the White House for a meeting. The coal presidents agreed to come but refused to negotiate. When Mitchell emerged from the meeting, he told the press that the coal-company presidents yelled at him for an hour. They can shout all they want, he said, but *the strike cannot be broken.* The only thing left to do was to send in the entire National Guard, which the governor did in early October. Gobin kept the Fourteenth Regiment in Mahanoy City and sent the Thirteenth to Olyphant, near Scranton. Two battalions of the Ninth Regiment marched to Plymouth and the rest set up camp near the Coxe Bros. & Co. Drifton colliery. The First Regiment rode into Hazleton with a battery of field artillery. Gobin sent field artillery to New Philadelphia, Minersville, and Tamaqua. All units had Gatling guns capable of firing ten rounds a second. The Eighth camped at Old Forge and the Fourth Regiment occupied a farm between Mt. Carmel and Shamokin. Nearly two thousand strikers lined the streets with their backs to the road when the troops came through town. By mid-October, more than ten thousand infantry, artillery, and cavalry troops had been activated. Gobin moved his headquarters from Shenandoah to Wilkes-Barre, leaving his tents at Columbia Park for the Eighteenth Regiment, which brought field artillery to Shenandoah. We're here for the purpose of protecting the non-union men, said the general, but there weren't many nonunion men left to protect.

Roosevelt called Mitchell and the mine owners back to Washington, but once again the coal companies refused to negotiate. They called the union a monopoly, and the strike a constraint on interstate trade. They said they'd come to Washington only if Roosevelt invoked the Sherman Act and sent in the troops. Go ahead, said the union. If all the troops in the United States were brought here, they could not force the men back to work. We'll outlast them too. Rumors began to spread that the coal companies were on the verge of waving the white flag. For what other reason would J. P. Morgan hold secret meetings in a yacht anchored off a westside New York dock? Why else would the publicity hound George Baer start ducking into side doors instead of talking to the press? Why else would John Mitchell tell the press that Morgan was friendly to organized labor? The miners held their breath, hoping for an end, thankful they'd survived it, and wondering what came next.

CHAPTER SIX

THE JEDDO EVICTIONS

When the strike began, George Bear convinced the other coal presidents to take a hard line with the strikers. A miners' union would be too great a threat, he told them. Even just acknowledging the UMW and Mitchell as the legitimate representatives of the coal miners would be disastrous. Mitchell will appoint himself *dictator of the coal business.* They'll determine wages and working conditions, decide who gets hired and who gets fired, and they'll claim law on their side when they do it. *We will not surrender,* they all said publicly. But by mid-October, five months into the strike, all the Coal and Iron Police and National Guard had succeeded in doing was hardening the resolve of the union. The coal companies had exhausted every tactic. When the scabs began joining the ranks of the strikers and Roosevelt rejected every demand for federal troops, the coal presidents finally agreed, secretly at first, to binding arbitration. They told Roosevelt they would only agree if the miners first returned to work, and even then, they would not formally negotiate with the union. The UMW could not be a party to the arbitration. And while they were willing to have Mitchell participate in the arbitration, he *could not appear on record as President of the United Mine Workers.*

Mitchell quickly agreed to their demands. The United Mine Workers of America would only be referred to as *the organization* during the hearings, not the United Mine Workers. And he would participate as the miners' spokesman, not their union president. When the deal went public, the American Federation of Labor celebrated it. Samuel Gompers called it splendid. Mother Jones, on the other hand, called it a trap. Why even consider it? *They know they're beaten.* Give them nothing. *Why walk into the House of Victory through the backdoor?* Have we not learned from the mistakes we made in 1900, when the operators offered a 10 percent raise but refused to recognize the union or even sign a contract? When that strike ended, the miners returned to work to find inflated prices in the company stores, eviction notices on shanty doors, the names of union leaders on the blacklists, scabs in all the best chambers and breasts, and the same excessive docking as always. The only miners who did better after the strike of 1900 were the snitches and scabs who crossed the picket line during it. What's to stop them from doing it again? We should dictate the terms. No, this time it's different, promised Mitchell. *I am informed through intermediaries the operators are inclined to be fair.*

Every local sent a delegate to a special convention in Wilkes-Barre to vote on the arbitration plan. Drum corps and union bands filled the streets in front of the Nesbitt theater on the day of the convention. The delegates entered the hall to the sound of a Mount Carmel miner, backed by a full orchestra, singing *The Strike That We Have Won*, an original composition he wrote special for the day. The doorkeepers threw open the doors and abandoned their posts—no reason to keep it a secret. The press and public rushed in to watch the deliberations, nearly outnumbering the miners. Mitchell took the stage to loud applause. *We recognize the right of capital to consolidate, but we demand and shall assert the same privileges for those who toil. Labor deserves the first consideration.* Yes, fine, but will we get our jobs back? Will we stand by the firemen and pumpmen who stood by us? Will there be a blacklist? *Some might not get their old places back and some might not be rehired at all*, said Mitchell. *But we knew the risks going in. No battle was ever fought that didn't claim some victims. Sacrifices must be made.* After two hours of discussion, and with Mitchell's recommendation, the delegates voted unanimously to accept the arbitration plan. Mitchell walked out of the hall and told a fairy tale to the press. *I earnestly hope and firmly believe that both labor and capital have learned from the miners' strike lessons which will enable them to adopt peaceful, humane, business methods of adjusting wage differences in the future.*

In the days that followed, Jeddo and Freeland miners found notices from G. B. Markle and Co. posted to trees and fences on the road to the collieries: *All men desiring to work for us are hereby notified to make application at our office at Jeddo, Penna., and to bring with them the brass checks we had heretofore issued.* The miners who showed up were told to hand over their brass checks and answer a few questions. *What's your age? What's your nationality? Married or single? Do you live in a company home? Did you work for us before? Will you abide by the decision of the arbitration commission*? While they gave their answers to one foreman, another searched the company roster for the name that corresponded to the number on their brass check, then cross-checked it against the company blacklist. Charlie Helferty, president of a union local, was turned away. Why? he asked. *Criminal acts.* No job for Charles Jacquott either. What reason? Because *you licked some parties in Freeland.* Same for Paul Dunleavy, treasurer of the Jeddo local, who spent thirty years working for Markle. *You'll never work for the company again.* Frank Ray, president of one of the union locals, who'd worked thirteen years in the mines, was also fired. *Could I at least get a recommendation so I can find another job?* No, said Sydney Williams, Markle's mine superintendent. Only Mr. Markle can do that. Henry Shovlin, outspoken Hazleton convention delegate, and Henry Coll, who lost an eye and walked with a limp after nineteen years of mining, were also turned away. Half-dead Jimmy Gallagher was told he'd never work again. Same for Andrew Hannik and Anthony Kamjuck. No job for John Gimshock, Joe Popucum, John Nohie, Charles Keenan. All were turned away.

When the fired miners told their district president Thomas Duffy about the blacklist, he told them they weren't alone and he'd received reports from other collieries about similar conditions. All the engineers, pumpmen, and firemen everywhere were being told their jobs had been filled. At Pardee's Cranberry colliery, returning strikers were told to sign a pledge if they wanted their jobs back: *As a condition precedent to my employment at A. Pardee & Co. I do hereby solemnly promise not to interfere with or molest in any way nay non-union men or any other men now at work or who may have worked during the strike, or who may work hereafter for my employers, and I do further agree to work with them as with any other employees.* Duffy ordered the miners out of the mine and into the streets, where they picketed all the roads that led to Markle's collieries. Markle sent word to Duffy that there wasn't a blacklist. He just wanted *to personally consider these men's cases before deciding whether they would be taken back or not.* Duffy sent a committee, and they told Markle *we went out in a body and we'll return in a body.* Markle refused, telling Duffy he didn't recognize his authority. On Friday, October 24, just days before the official start of the arbitration commission, Markle agreed to meet with a smaller committee of three union miners to discuss the matter. *There are certain men who can never return to work on this property,* he told them. *Not account of their being United Mine Workers, but on account of their individual acts.* What acts? they asked, but Markle wouldn't say. I can't tell you. *It might expose certain men to the revenge which we know would follow.*

Duffy organized a meeting to discuss their options. So many miners showed up that the union hall couldn't hold them, so they built a stage in a dirt lot and held the meeting outdoors instead. Gallagher spoke first and implored the miners to return to work. We're no martyrs, he said. This is just the price we pay. *There never was a victory yet without somebody getting lost.* We can't hold 2,500 men out of work just to protect a dozen. But the miners wouldn't hear it. The arbitration hearings haven't even begun. Why should they have the right to fire anyone when we won the strike? *We go back in a body or not at all.* Markle complained about the meeting in a telegram to Carrol Wright. *Our men have not returned to work. They are not acting in conformity with the conditions upon which your Commission was created. Picket lines had been thrown out, threats and intimidations were being made.* He made vague references about falsehoods and false impressions. He promised Wright he'd take all the men back excepting a few who have been party to criminal actions. Mitchell refused to intervene, worried the conflict might derail the arbitration. He ordered the miners back to the mines.

With the resumption of mining, Markle began evicting the blacklisted miners. On Monday, October 27, the day the arbitration hearings began in Washington, his colliery police chief, Gottlieb Filler, went door-to-door in Jeddo posting eviction notices on front doors. When the miners found them, they tore them down and brought them to Duffy, who gave them to the union lawyer D. J. McCarthy, who asked the miners for copies of their leases. Not one of them had a copy. Some had never even seen one. Gallagher said he could hardly remember signing one, it was too long ago. I've lived there ever *since I came to the country* and only vaguely remember *signing a hand-written piece of paper,* but I don't know what it said because I don't read. The thing I remember is that the house had no locks. *There wasn't a key. It was open and ghosts and everything were in there.*

McCarthy sent the miners to get copies of their lease, but Markle's clerk refused to provide them. *It's not permitted,* he told them. *A tenant cannot have a copy of the lease.* McCarthy finally found a copy on Thursday, and he showed it to the Luzerne County sheriff. Look, he said, Markle added a clause to the standard language that makes it easier for him to evict these men. These are *cut-throat agreements,* not leases. Has Markle delivered writs of eviction yet? he asked. No, said the sheriff, who claimed to be unaware of any upcoming evictions. *I've prepared an application to the court to open up the judgment so the miners can defend themselves,* but this won't keep them in their houses unless I make an application to one of the judges before the men are turned out. Will you warn me if you hear anything? The sheriff promised he would. I hate evicting miners. *It's such an unpleasant thing to do.* I'll do *anything to help prevent them from being ejected.* You can trust me. *I'm in sympathy with these men.*

But a week later and without warning, the sheriff marched into Jeddo with a handful of eviction writs accompanied by three Markle superintendents, a posse of Coal and Iron Police, and two companies of National Guard soldiers. *What could I do?* he would say later. *I was compelled.*

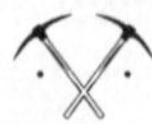

The mine patches were remote company towns built near breakers and cut off from the world. They were small villages of wood-framed structures clad with warped hemlock and covered in cheap weather stripping. Interior walls were often left unplastered and some had no ceilings or battens. Each shanty faced a dirt street that led to the colliery in one direction and the company store in the other. Nearly every coal company had them. The Philadelphia and Reading Coal and Iron Co. rented 2,000 shanties to miners for two dollars a month. The Lehigh Coal Co. rented out 700. Lehigh and Wilkes-Barre leased 450. Coxe Bros. & Co. rented out 879. Van Wickle leased 300. Markle rented more than 500 shanties for fifteen cents a day. The

Jeddo shanties were two-story buildings, sixteen feet by sixteen feet square. Each had two small rooms on the first floor and two more on the second. They came with unfinished third-floor garrets and shallow dirt cellars. A rough kitchen shack was attached to the back for summertime use.

Henry and Mary Coll were asleep when the Jeddo evictions began, kept in bed by sickness and lack of work. His legs had never healed from that runaway coal car in '93. He still had the scars from when a cop gave him a beating in '96. He suffered constant headaches from when a roof fell on him in '99 and fractured his skull. Mary, his wife, lay beside him, complaining of throat trouble that wouldn't improve. Her mother lay in another bed in another room, *sick and blind besides,* with barely enough strength to make her way around the house *groping two inches at a time.* Henry's son James lay in the last bed next to the two young orphans whom Henry and Mary had recently taken in. The knock came just after dawn and when Henry opened the door, he found the sheriff standing in front of a squad of cops holding papers in his hands. *You got a six-days' notice. Now's two days more. You have the right to get out.* But we got no place to go, Henry protested. I need a day at least to find a place. No, said the sheriff. *You had ample time.* Henry said something about Coxe Bros. giving ten days' warning. This isn't Coxe Bros. *This is different papers*, said the sheriff. But Mary's sick, he said, and we got an old-timer upstairs. The sheriff turned and walked back to discuss the issue with a lawyer standing in the street. *They're stalling*, the lawyer told him. *They want to get out an injunction and stop the proceedings.* There can be no reprieve. The sheriff walked back to Henry and told him he *cannot have five minutes now.* When Henry kept pleading, the sheriff turned and made a signal to the cops. They moved forward as one, pushing past Henry and into the house. One crew began hauling out small tables, chairs, an oil lamp, and blankets, dumping everything in a pile in the street. Two cops climbed the stairs and came down carrying Mary's mother on a mattress; four others helped haul her through the door and out to the street. By then Mary was standing in a drizzling rain scrambling to keep her clothes and furniture out of the mud. Children trying to be helpful dragged barrels and boxes to her, but she couldn't keep up. At the other end of the street, a line of soldiers stood along a fence line, watching silently. The sound of loud and angry talking brought people into the street. They stood in twos and threes and watched the cops drag heavy furniture from the Coll house, tear curtains from windows, and dump armfuls of belongings into piles that grew so large it blocked the narrow dirt street. Mary turned to Henry and told him to go find a house in Hazleton, or anywhere Markle didn't own everything. So this is how it ends, thought Henry, as he made his way to Hazleton. And he thought to himself, So this is how it ends. *I always knew we was doomed.*

When the cops were done with the Colls, they moved on to the next house, where Paul Dunleavy, standing on his small front porch, was waiting for them. *This is very sudden, ain't it?* Yes, said the sheriff, *it is kind of sudden.* Listen, Paul said, *I'm in a pretty bad fix here. Both of the old people are sick, have been ailing for three or four days, and the old gentlemen in particular. I would like if you could give me until tomorrow morning. I am ready to go to Hazleton now and I'll try all in my power to get a house.* The sheriff just looked at him for a few seconds and then said, *Paul, you have to get out in five minutes.* The cops were working quickly now, laughing and joking as they went. A union photographer arrived from Hazleton and began taking pictures of the cops and the growing piles of furniture. An artist set up an easel and sketched scenes of cops dumping Dunleavy's things on the street. Children grabbed toys from the pile to keep them out of the rain. Girls on their way to silk mills stopped and consoled girls being evicted. Dunleavy's seven-year-old son, who worked for Markle as a breaker boy, ran out of the house with an American flag and planted it defiantly on the growing pile of furniture in the street, the only time all day anyone cheered.

Henry Shovlin was next. *Good morning, Henry. Do you know who I am? I suppose I do,* said Henry. *Any sparings to give? No,* said the sheriff. *Nothing whatsoever.* Can I *at least have till the afternoon. Tomorrow would be even better. It'd give me a chance to get another place.* No, said the sheriff, *You don't get two minutes. These men are waiting outside your door ready to go to work.* Henry stepped aside and watched them go in and out, carrying beds and chairs, hauling out the stove, dragging sixty bushels of potatoes from the cellar, piling everything on the street.

It went on like this all day. They threw Helferty out of his house and then Jacquott too. The cops pulled seven barrels of sauerkraut and three hogsheads from Gimshock's cellar. By the time they reached Half-dead Jimmy Gallagher's house, the cops were taunting and teasing the miners, enjoying themselves. They called Gallagher *Granny* as they pushed him out of the way. *If I was fit to walk they would have throwed me out alongside it all.* Gallagher, who hadn't been paid in nearly eighteen years, couldn't afford a trolley ride into Hazleton. He walked seven miles in the rain to look for a new house, pausing at Markle's Jeddo office on the way. He saw Charlie Helferty arguing with John Markle. *Mr. Markle, what did you throw me out for? What did I do?* he asked. *I put you out for criminal acts,* Markle told him. Gallagher stepped in front of Helferty and looked Markle in the eye. *I known you from boyhood when you wore a little short pair of pants. Tell me, John, what do you throw me out for? Like all the rest,* said Markle. *Criminal acts. When is it I ever did those things?* Gallagher asked. *Your memory must be short, Jim. No,* said Gallagher. *My memory's not short. To my knowledge I never hurted man, woman, or child in my life, therefore where is my criminal acts?*

Back in Jeddo, Charles Keenan, Joseph Popucum, and Mike Cushma watched as the cops turned their homes inside out, one after the other. It was nearly afternoon by the time the police broke down Andrew Hannik's door. I can't move, protested Hannik in halting English. My wife's in bad shape. *Why didn't you move out when the time was up to move, when you got your notice?* asked the sheriff. I tried, *but I couldn't find a house.* The sheriff shook his head. *How will you feel now when I have to throw you out in the street?* What's the point of arguing? thought Hannik. *Do as you please. Do as you like.*

Henry Coll got back to Jeddo just as Hannik was being evicted. He went looking for Mary and found her at a neighbor's house exhausted, her wet hair flattened against her head, her voice even hoarser than before. The cops hauled our things out to the public highway, she told him, and dumped everything in the mud by the side of the road. Stay in Jeddo and keep out of the rain, he told her. I'll haul everything to Hazleton. When Henry arrived at the new house, he found that he couldn't fit the large furniture through the small, front door, so he tore out a side window and wrestled their things into the house until he was exhausted. He couldn't lift the stove by himself, so he left it in the yard and rode back to Jeddo to collect Mary and the children. They slept that night under damp blankets in a cold room huddled together on muddy mattresses.

In the morning, shivering, Mary said, for God's sake, Henry, *go to Paul Dunleavy's and get help.* I need an ambulance. Where would it take you? he asked. *You can't go to the Miners' hospital.* And what's the point of calling the doctor? he thought. *I did not have no money to get a doctor with.* Instead he helped her to her feet and walked her around the house, warming her in his arms. He spent the next few days looking for a house with a stove while Mary and the children stayed with a miner's family in Hazleton. The rest and warmth improved her condition, and when she was able to walk again, she went to see the doctor, who gave her a bottle of medicine and told her to stay warm and get rest. He promised to come check on her in a couple days. Henry tried to give him a dollar, but the doctor wouldn't take it. *You people was evicted. You need it more than I do.*

It took Henry a week to find a house that had a stove and that they could afford. By then Mary looked better, he thought, or at least *did not appear to be anyways serious or near death.* Mary's cough hadn't gone away, but at least they had a warm house and dry bedding. But then on an early December night, as they *lay down at half-past* ten to go to sleep, she asked him for her medicine. Later, when he would think of this moment, he would be reminded of the breathlessness in her voice and the wide-eyed look on her face when she pointed to the medicine on the table. *I'm choking. It might give me a little breath*, she gasped. Henry grabbed the bottle but before he could open it, Mary sprang up in the bed, as if pulled by some invisible force. When he turned to look at her, he saw that her face was flushed bright red and her hands were gripping her neck. He dropped the bottle and took her into his arms and could feel her body tremble and tighten. He yelled and screamed, or at least must have, he didn't remember doing it. The sound of the screaming sent the children running from the house. They tumbled out the door and startled a Polish man who was walking past. Thinking there must be a fire, the man ran into the house. I thought I heard screaming, he explained, but all he found was Mary and Henry on the bed in each other's arms. What was the screaming for? the man asked. *I suppose it was just the noise I made*, Henry said, *when I seen she was dying.*

CHAPTER SEVEN

SHOW US THE LUNG OF A MINER

The independent operators of the Lehigh valley refuse to submit to arbitration or even participate in the hearings. The only way to deal with these *outlaws*, says John Markle to President Roosevelt, *is by the strong arm of the military at your command.* J. P. Morgan's cartel agrees to participate but refuses to call it an arbitration. *This is an investigation by a commission,* they say, and nothing more. We make no concessions to the union, a spokesman explains. *It's a concession to humanity,* one coal president calls it, not the miners' union. Once the union votes for the arbitration plan, the coal companies announce they will only participate if Roosevelt puts a military man on the commission; also a coal engineer, a coal dealer, no labor organizers, and no bleeding hearts. Roosevelt agrees and appoints Thomas H. Watkins, a former independent coal operator from Scranton, Brigadier General John M. Wilson, of the Army's engineer corps, and E. W. Parker, the part-time editor of an industry factsheet who works as a mining engineer in the government's Coal Division. At J. P. Morgan's personal request, he appoints former Delaware senator Judge George Gray to the commission. When Mitchell sees the roster, he threatens to withdraw from the arbitration, so Roosevelt adds E. E. Clark, grand chief of the Order of Railway Conductors, and the Illinois bishop John L. Spalding,

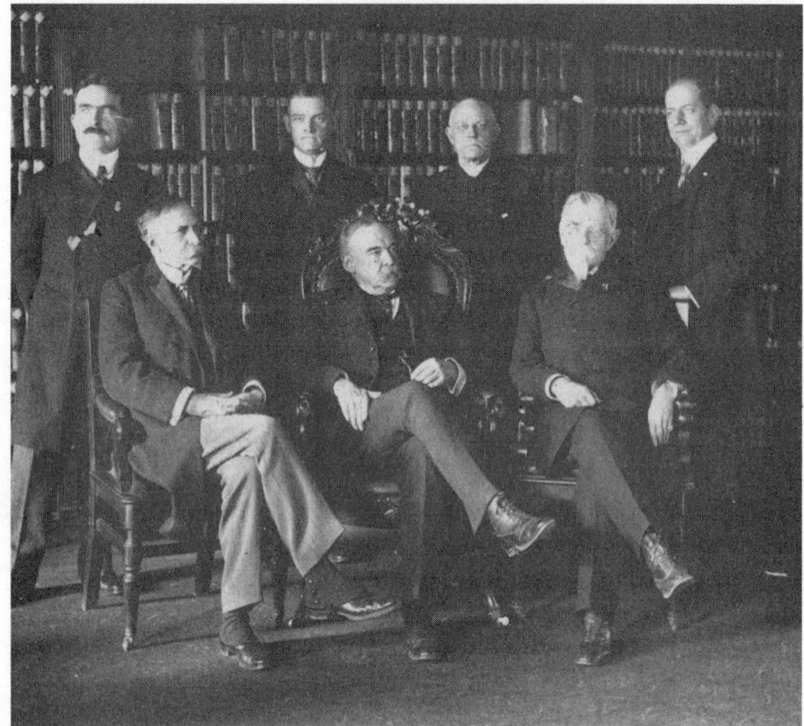

The Anthracite Coal Strike Commission. Front row, left to right: Labor Commissioner Carroll Wright, Judge George Gray, Brigadier General John M. Wilson; back row, left to right: Thomas H. Watkins, E. E. Clark, Bishop John L. Spalding, E. W. Parker. Courtesy: Library of Congress.

both of whom had openly supported the mine workers during the strike.

The coal companies can't agree on a shared defense, so every company sends its own team of lawyers and accountants to the commission hearings. Mitchell hires Clarence Darrow to represent the mine workers. Though not yet the national celebrity he would later become after the Scopes Trial, he is well known among union miners for his work representing Eugene V. Debs in the witch hunt that followed the 1894 Pullman porter strike. The hearings open in Washington, DC, in late October, just days after the miners return to work and before the Jeddo evictions begin. Judge Gray, appointed the commission's chairman, orders the coal companies to provide accurate wage data for all their employees. When the lawyers say it will take weeks to compile the information, the commission suspends the hearings and takes a fact-finding tour of the anthracite fields. They tour washeries and breakers and visit mine patches and miners' homes. When they arrive in Drifton on the first of November, L. C. Smith greets them at the train station. *We're in favor of taking back the old employees in a body*, he tells them, reading from a prepared statement, but we don't need as many as we did before the strike, what with all the *labor-saving machinery* we've installed. From Drifton the commissioners travel to Jeddo, where John Markle and Sydney Williams take them on a drive-by tour of the shops, the breaker, and the homes of the soon-to-be-evicted miners. From there they go to Hazleton, where they smoke cigars with Frank Pardee in the parlor of the Central Hotel, and finally to Audenried to take a tour of a mine, which almost doesn't happen when the commissioners arrive to find an agitated crowd of women and children waiting for them at the mouth of the slope. It takes an hour to convince the crowd that there hasn't been an explosion in the mine, that none of the commissioners are mine inspectors, and that all of their husbands and fathers are still alive.

The commission reconvenes the hearings in Scranton on November 14, and Darrow calls John Mitchell to the stand to present the union's demands. Hard-rock mining is no normal job, he explains. A miner starts in the breaker as a little boy, *works his way up, step by step*, until he becomes a contract miner. The mine owners say otherwise, but we all know this is a job that *requires an unusually high degree of skill*. What's the reward for all that experience and skill? A steady decline in health and wages, that's what. After a lifetime working his way up to become a contract miner, he *works his way back down. You'll find many old men who have been forced, after a lifetime of unremitting toil, to return to the breaker where they worked as a boy, there to earn a pittance barely sufficient to keep body and soul together.* Every job in a mine is *dangerous work. Each day the anthracite coal mines are in operation*, you can be sure that two miners will be killed, some days more, *and three times as many are maimed.* This job isn't just dangerous, *it's extra-hazardous and therefore* the miners should *be especially well paid for their laborious and dangerous calling.* But the owners pay the miners as if they have no skill, as if anyone could do this job. He works knee-deep in water, crouching and bending day after day, *breathing powder, smoke, foul air* year after year. And even if the miner does it well, even *if he escapes death or injury by falls of rock or coal*, his fate is sealed. *He cannot escape attacks of miners' asthma.* We demand a 20 percent wage increase and a nine-hour day. We demand to be *paid by the weight.* We demand that the miners' ton be abolished. *A ton should be twenty-two hundred and forty pounds, not 3,190 pounds.* And *we demand a trade agreement that includes a grievance procedure.* The miner

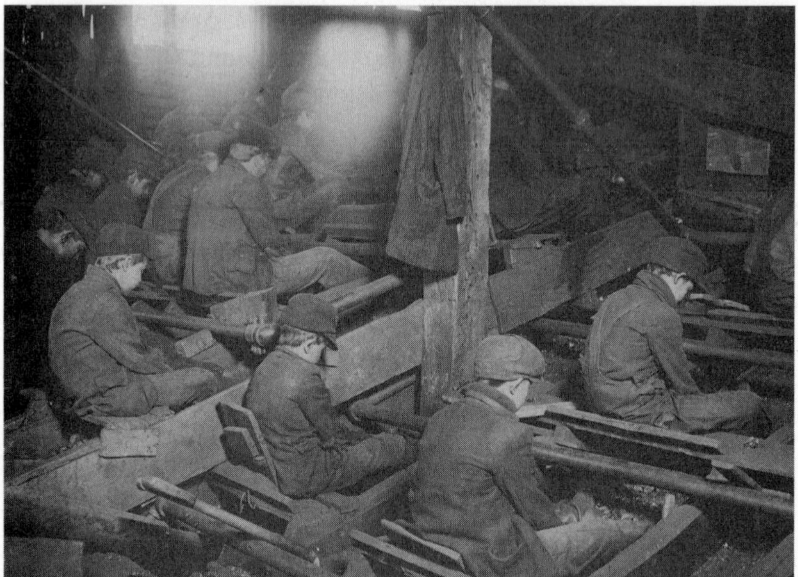

The boys in the Pittston breaker. Courtesy: Library of Congress.

deserves better than what he gets. Don't forget what these miners do and what their labor gives us. Our civilization depends on the labor of *those who enter the bowels of the earth* and set *in motion the wheels of commerce.*

After Mitchell, miner after miner takes the stand and tells harrowing stories of dangerous working conditions, of powder smoke so thick they can't see their hands in front of their faces, of methane so bad they stagger out of the mine. Darrow puts children on the stand who describe working ten or more hours a day, six days a week, in dusty breakers where the coal comes careening down metal chutes. We work hunched over on wooden benches, they testify, sitting shoulder to shoulder, our chapped hands plunged into black, freezing water, separating slate from coal. Hands mangled by machinery, bodies crushed by gears. They describe being brought into the mine as toddlers by fathers who need candles kept lit. Seventeen-year-old Mike Baker describes picking slate from coal six days a week, fourteen-hours a day, at barely more than five cents an hour. Darrow asks if he ever gets *clubbed by the slate picker boss.*

Yes sir, I got clubbed often.
Does he hurt you when he clubs you?
Yes, sir.
Does he ever kick you?
Yes, sir.
And swear at you?
Yes sir.
What do you mean by clubbing?
He clubs me with a stick.
How big a stick?
About so long (indicating about three feet)
How often does that happen, nearly every night?
Yes, sir.

Twelve-year-old Andrew Chippie describes bosses pulling his ears to make him work faster and being forced to work in the mines to pay off a dead father's debt. Darrow asks him how much he is paid.

I don't get no money.
How do you get by then?
My mother takes in boarders.

The foremen and superintendents make a show of condemning child labor and then, under cross-examination, admit that they hire boys twelve and younger for the breakers and as young as thirteen for the mines. If you condemn it, why do you do it? It's customary *through the coalfield, an old custom kept up.* But you claim the boys are hard to handle and too young besides, so *why won't your company just stop hiring them*? It's impossible. *So long as others did it, we certainly would have to do the same thing.* It just isn't *feasible* to abolish child labor when everyone else does it, what with our shareholder obligations based on standard industry practices.

Miners testify to all the ways the mine owners undercut their wages. The contractors hire inexperienced mine laborers to drive columnways and shafts and then pocket half their wages. They give lengthy testimony about how Markle controls the labor process through his two-tiered powder price. Most miners conserve their powder to save on the expense and to limit their exposure to smoke, but this produces smaller, less valuable sizes of coal. So Markle doubled the price of powder. If the miners wanted the old price, they had to increase the amount of powder they used. They were forced to drill more holes in the dark, pack more powder into the earth, and fire larger and more frequent explosions, which meant working longer in smoke-filled chambers held up by timbers rattled by the blasts.

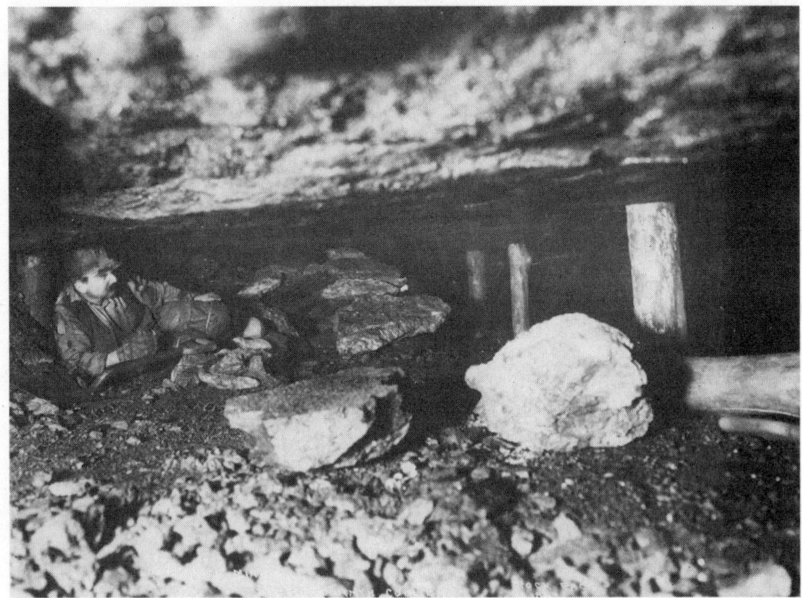
A miner working a thirty-six inch breast. Courtesy: Indiana University of Pennsylvania Special Collections and University Archive

Darrow asks the miners to describe their working conditions, and they testify about breasts and chambers so tight they spend half their lives on their knees, or bent over, or lying on their backs in water picking at coal. They are asked the cause of all the black and blue spots and cuts on their faces and hands, and they explain that it's the earth that came *flying from the pick-point* of every swing of the axe that did it. Each swing produces a small explosion of coal *striking on the hand and face* and piercing the skin. Eventually the black and blue marks cover every inch of a man's face and hands until he looks twice his age, *all cut and disfigured.* Coal once buried in the earth is now buried in them.

Darrow calls poor house doctors to the stand who estimate that upward of 70 or 80 percent of their patients are former miners. Miners who have *all become anemic; whose blood is impoverished; ninety percent* of whom suffer from *some form of rheumatism, neuralgia, asthma.* Their lungs turn so black they look like *a chunk of anthracite coal.* Miners say that when they try to get themselves checked into hospitals they are turned away because the hospitals don't have enough beds to treat chronic cases. The doctors tell stories of miners who suffer violent paroxysms of coughing and choking from inhaling carbon dioxide and methane-poisoned air. Their lips turn blue. Their bodies develop a gaunt, emaciated appearance, which causes them to walk with a dull, haggard, shuffling gait. Every labored breath seems surely their last.

Eventually, their stories merge into a kind of collective story, a common tale of a hard-rock miner's hard-luck life. He starts as a boy picking slate all day in the breaker and skipping school at night. At thirteen he is promoted into the mines, where he spends years deep underground, opening and closing the massive doors that control the mine's ventilation. He gets a job as a muledriver delivering cars to miners for a few pennies an hour. His father is killed, or disappears, or is blacklisted. He is promoted to laborer so he can pay his dead father's debts and shovels coal for sixty cents a car. He loses a finger to a squib, an eye to smoke. Sees a man lose an arm to a runaway coal car. He becomes a certified miner in his late twenties, gets married, is pinned between a prop and a runaway coal car, and spends a month in the hospital, emerging with a limp. He lives in a shanty where his children drink water from a creek fouled by mine waste and sewage, and he watches with alarm as red rashes and raised welts appear on their abdomens. He is shot by a cop during a strike. A daughter dies in a squib factory explosion. Ailments accumulate as he ages. Methane poisons his blood. Coal dust colonizes his lungs. He becomes known by the sound of his cough. He looks seventy when he turns fifty. His face becomes so disfigured by cuts and burns that people look away when they see him. When he can't keep up the pace any longer, a foreman sends him to the same breaker he worked as a boy. A doctor diagnoses him with melancholy, predicts dementia, finds him a bed in the alms-house, where he dies from causes so numerous no doctor is certain what killed him.

Mining coal doesn't just turn the earth inside out, it turns the miner inside out too. Darrow puts doctors and coroners on the stand, and one brings a half-dozen samples of lungs with him. *Have you here with you any samples showing just the condition of a miner's lung?* asks Darrow. *I have*, the doctor replies. *We would like to have you show them*, Darrow says. The chairman gasps. *A miner's lung?* he says. Yes, says Darrow, *a miner's lung, as compared with the normal lung.* The doctor walks to a table that holds jars of lungs and begins his show-and-tell, pulling them out one by one, placing them on the table. *There is a normal lung*, he says, pointing to the one nearest the commissioners. *Which one?* asks the chairman. T*he one right up against the jar*, he says, pointing to something that looks like a pale-red, oval-shaped, half-inflated balloon. *That's the normal lung, is it?* asks Darrow. *As nearly normal as we get*, says the doctor. *Now*, says Darrow, *show us the lung of a miner.* The doctor has his pick. *Here's one showing an early stage*, he says, pointing to a hard, brown-and-red disk covered in black spots. *And there are others*, he says, opening his hands to indicate the whole table. These show *different stages of the coal miner's lungs*, he tells them. *Is that second one a miner's lung?* asks Commissioner Parker, the mining engineer. *Yes*, says the doctor, pointing to a hard, flat disc that looks painted black. *All those black ones are miner's lungs?* asks Darrow, pointing at a table of miners' lungs so charred they look as though pulled from a blast furnace. Yes, sir, says the doctor. The coal dust accumulates in a miner's lungs and eventually causes uncontrollable *spasmodic contractions of the muscular layers of these little bronchial tubes*. This coal dust so saturates their *lungs the miners cough up sputum so black you could write with it. You could use it for ink*. Cysts form in their lungs and collapse the vesicles, which eventually turns the entire lung into a hardened mass of fibrous tissue. The miner's own lungs rob him of breath and eventually asphyxiate him. The chairman wants to know if a miner's lung sinks in water. Yes, says the doctor. *Parts of them will.* The lawyer for the mine owners wants to know if the table full of blackened lungs could also be considered evidence of *the healthfulness of mining. No,* says the doctor, it could not. Bishop Spalding wants to know if the blackest-looking lungs on the table *were the lungs of colored men. No, sir, I think not,* says the doctor, to the laughter of the commissioners.

When the hearings move to Philadelphia in January, the coal-company lawyers put statisticians, paymasters, and accountants on the stand, all of whom say they've run the numbers and have found that miners are paid above their worth and get more than they deserve. We can think of no other job that requires *so little special training or skill,* so little effort and *physical energy,* so *little risk of injury,* and takes up *so small a portion of the working day,* and yet is so *liberally compensated in wages, as the work of the anthracite miner.* These miners work a few months out of a year and yet make thousands of dollars, they exclaim. Our wage lists show it. Darrow puts miners on the stand to rebut their testimony. The numbers are accurate, says Daniel Evans. I did make $1,580 in 1901. But *I was working two miners and two laborers* for part of the year and *three-handed—two laborers and one man*—the rest. You say you split $1,580 among all those men? Darrow asks. Yes, he says. *We put the bulk of the money together and paid both laborers out to it, and then divided up what was left.* Same was true for Shadrach Lewis, who the accountants say made around $1,900 in 1901. I worked with another miner, he explains, and two laborers. What did you do with the wages they paid you? *Divided it between him and I and paid the other boys,* he explains. *About how much did you get out of this $1,900 yourself after paying everything? I got $661.58.* Frank Richards cleared $2,269.20 in 1900. But after paying laborers and after the colliery *deducted all expenses, I had about $750.* These wage data are useless, complains Darrow. The coal companies know the contract miners pay their own laborers, but they pass the data off as if they're the wages of one man. Is it the job of a statistician *to present misleading figures*?

The coal companies put little girls on the stand and ask them why they work in the silk mills when their fathers make so much money. Darrow recalls John Demko to the stand, whose daughter works the mills. *The Company has furnished a schedule which was given out here yesterday*, Darrow says. It claimed that you earned or received $1,400. Through an interpreter, Demko explains that he worked with two other miners and two laborers. My butty and me *paid the laborers what would come to them and whatever was left we divided between ourselves, the miners.* Darrow asks him to tell the commissioners why his daughter must work the mill. *Well, gentlemens, I was in bad position. I got six small children buried inside of five years, and my wife was in asylum for pretty near two years. Then I have five to keep same time she was away, you know. I made decent money, but I was very bad with the debt in the store, so they sent the girl to the mill to help me pay the debts.* She works overnight, he says. What could I do?

Judge Gray scolds the company lawyers. Your misleading data *shake our faith* in your honesty. When you *give a miner's wages*, he demands, make sure it's *really what he received himself.* Yes, sir, say the lawyers, and they return a week later with new wage tables that describe the average wage rates of what they call *composite* miners. Why not just average the actual wages of your actual miners and provide that? asks Darrow. We can't, they say. We don't know who's who. We can't keep track of the Poles and Hungarians. *They change from one place to another. They go from one colliery to another. They will work in one part of the mines under one name, and we will find probably the same man in another part of the mines with perhaps a slight difference in names, so that it is impossible to tell whether it is the identical man. There are so many of them it was found that the task was almost impossible.* Also, the men quit so often and in such great numbers that average wages aren't representative. Some miners work only ten days and then disappear. Some come and go and work only thirty days in a year. What's important is the average, annual wage of a hypothetical miner who worked every day and made the best wages possible. Darrow objects. These aren't *real earnings,* he says. No one actually made this money. These are hypothetical *possible earnings of impossible men.* What insight does this give us? One colliery submits wage tables that exclude all miners whose names they can't pronounce, which results in an average, annual wage greater than the actual wages of 96 percent of the company's miners. That's an interesting methodology, Darrow notes. *Like averaging the total earnings of a railroad president with the office boy.*

Darrow's mockery has little effect. The company lawyers continue to make unsubstantiated claims, which grow more ridiculous as the hearings progress. The wages may appear small, but it's not like the job requires *skill* or *intelligence.* If miners really wanted higher wages, they'd leave the coalfields, but instead they stay *for the scenery.* They *seem wedded to the place,* which you can't blame us for. Their hardships are their own fault. They could make more, but the union holds them back. They're lazy. *It's a well-known fact* they put their children to work in the mills and mines to support them *in their idleness.* They enter the mines and then *sit around and smoke.* If there is suffering, don't blame us. Blame it on *their intemperance.* The miners don't deserve higher wages. It's not like they're *American born and American bred men.* They make more here than in Europe. We pay good wages, for *foreigners.* They lack *habits of frugality* and waste their money on *whiskey* and *cigars* and extravagances such as *pianos and house organs.* There are saloons on every corner and *every house is a drinking place.* They get drunk on payday and disappear for days on end.

What's with the sociological obsession? Darrow asks. He is forced to call witnesses to the stand to vouch for a general absence of pianos in the coalfields. He calls doctors and priests who insist that the miners drink only as much as the next guy. He recalls scores of miners back to the stand to explain why they leave the mines early. It's not from laziness, they say. We leave early only when we are suffocated at the face and stagger out of the mines barely alive. The miner Thomas Powell shows the commissioners his glass eye. *I lost it owing to powder smoke,* he tells them. We make poor wages, they all explain, because the bosses pay poor wages. They put us in a poor place with a dirty vein where we *work hard like a dog* but make nothing. Or we fire a shot and when we sound the top coal, we hear the hollow sound that tells us we need timber to reinforce the roof, but the timber takes a week to arrive. Or they send us to rob pillars and the roof collapses. Or we fire a shot and pull coal from the face and then wait for cars that never come because the foreman gives them to his friends instead. Or the breaker shuts down, and the cars line up at the bottom of the shaft waiting to be hoisted. It's true, Darrow says. The miners themselves limit the number of cars they let other miners have. But do you see why they do it? *The miners have sought to regulate the crusts that have been thrown to them so that one man should not have a loaf while the other has nothing.* The lawyers counter by putting a superintendent on the stand who can testify to the way wages are determined. OK, Darrow says. How are wages determined?

I think the wages we are paying now are very reasonable.
How much do you think is a reasonable price per day?
The wages we are paying now are very reasonable.
What is that?
I cannot recall those figures.

Then why do you think they are reasonable?
Because we are paying them.

One company accountant submits tables that he claims show that the miners' wages are high, that mining is the *healthiest business in the world,* and that every other job in America is more dangerous. One testifies that tailors, art teachers, and even preachers die at a rate higher than miners. Darrow teases him and calls *him unqualified to teach kindergarten.* Half of all hard-rock miners who died in 1900, Darrow points out, died a violent death in the mines. How does that compare to preaching? Granted, Darrow concedes, it might be *dangerous to the congregation, but to the preacher?*

The coal companies have recommendations to make. The problem isn't low wages, insist the bosses, but recalcitrant miners. They call the Lattimer killers Ario Pardee Platt and Willard Young to the stand in late January 1903. These men have discovered a solution to the problem of recalcitrant miners. Explain to the commission what the Flying Squadron is, asks the attorney for the Lehigh Coal and Navigation Co. *It was a body of men,* Platt says, *policemen. If an attack was reported, they went to the assistance of the collier who wanted them.* Dedicated trains were always available, *night and day.* We established *posts and outposts,* he explains. Police always on duty. Every colliery was connected to the Flying Squadron by phone. They could be brought quickly to *any point* in the territory. The commissioners have their own questions. *Any toughs or bummers among your troopers?* asks the chairman. No, sir. *Only good, honest men,* Platt says. All with military and police experience. The results of the Flying Squadron are undeniable, claims the lawyer. It was a force of professional men, held to high standards, and because of it was *able practically to disperse all the mobs which gathered.* Their performance was *very encouraging indeed.* It proves *the value of a State constabulary.*

Platt charms the commissioners. When he says that only good men served on the Flying Squadron, the chairman enthusiastically agrees with him. And *you were one of them*, he says. Yes, I was, agrees Platt, and the courtroom breaks out in appreciative laughter. *Modesty always blushes*, Platt says to more laughter. Well, the chairman replies, *I think you are a pretty good sample* of the quality of police in the Flying Squadron. During cross-examination, Darrow's second chair, D. J. McCarthy, the lawyer for the evicted Jeddo miners, tries to impeach Platt's testimony by pointing out the many times the Flying Squadron incited riots and made arbitrary arrests. He reminds the commissioners that Platt played a role in the Lattimer Massacre.

You were in the disturbance at Lattimer?
I was at Lattimer. Tried and acquitted.
How many men were killed in that riot?
I don't know, that is past history, that is ancient.
Is it not a fact, Mr. Pardee, that a large number of men were killed there?
Yes, my recollection is it was 19. You know better than I do because you evidently keep it in mind.
How many were wounded?
I think that number was 39, wasn't it? I really forget.
These men were shot down by sheriff Martin's posse, were they not?
They were.
A great many of these men were shot in the back, were they not?
I don't know, I didn't make the medical examinations.
Mr. Platt, you were indicted and tried?
Yes, sir, and acquitted.
Among others, for the murder of these men?
That is right.
You were present during the trial?

I was, yes, sir.
You heard the testimony that a large number of these men were shot in the back?
I know it, I saw it on the ground.
You do know it?
I did know it, I know it now. I saw them, helped take care of them after they were shot, did my very best to—
Were these men that were shot down armed, Mr. Platt?
Well, I don't think that has any bearing.
You were there?
I am here and you are there. I don't know whether you are armed or not.
I was not at Lattimer.
I say I don't know whether you are armed or not.
Do you know whether they were armed or not?
I do not.
About how many men were in that crowd that you shot into?
The mob, do you mean?

When Platt's lawyer objects to McCarthy's line of questioning, Judge Gray orders McCarthy to drop it. *Lattimer has nothing to do with anything before us,* he says. Platt returns to his testimony on the Flying Squadron, explaining how it was organized, describing what weapons it had, recounting how it moved around the region, and extolling its virtues. The men were well-trained and well-behaved. *I was acquainted with all of them.* Platt says he was intimately involved in Flying Squadron operations. It was only through the constant vigilance of the Flying Squadron that disorder was suppressed. *It was their duty to protect the property night and day. They were officers of the law and performed their duty well.* Enough praise, McCarthy says. Let's talk specific examples.

Did the Flying Squadron make any arrests?
I don't know.
Do you know whether or not they ever gathered up some coal pickers and handcuffed them together and dragged them from Cresco to Hazleton?
All I know about that is what you just told me.
And the six men arrested at No. 6 on your property, or adjoining property on the Lehigh Valley?
No, sir, don't know anything about it.
And the men railroaded to Weatherly?
I know only what you told me.
Can you tell us about the time the Flying Squadron endeavored to precipitate a riot in Squire Bucklin's office?
No, I wasn't there, my duties were all at Cranberry.

It goes on like this until McCarthy asks whether Platt arrested miners without a warrant, at which point Platt, who previously claimed to know everything about the Flying Squadron, says he doesn't know much about it.

Do you know they arrested men without warrant?
No, I don't know that.
Will you say the Flying Squadron did not arrest men without warrants?
I say I don't know they did.
You do not know they did not?
I am trying to tell you with all the candor possible. I know nothing about their doings at all.

Willard Young takes the stand next and describes the creation of the Flying Squadron as an effort to fix all that was bad with private police. We raised standards and recruited carefully. We hired men with military experience, and they pledged their loyalty to the public good. The Flying Squadron demonstrated that police can serve as an effective deterrent to crime and disorder. He describes the Flying Squadron as the model for a new state constabulary. Our troopers weren't allowed to drink, Young explains. We didn't come in guns first, we dispersed crowds without violence, made arrests without ever firing a shot. *The upshot of all this,* summarizes the lawyer, *is that by exercising care in the selection of your men, and having control over them, you were able to disperse every mob without any violence.* One commissioner asks Young if the strike would have been worse if not for the Flying Squadron. Yes, replies Young. We found ourselves *most decidedly* under *a reign of terror* during this strike and *yet, the Flying Squadron resolved every dispute without the use of violence.*

The hearings come to an end in mid-February, after nearly six hundred witnesses and more than three months of testimony. The commissioners return to Washington, DC, and deliberate in private for more than month. When they emerge with their report on March 21, every coalfield newspaper publishes their findings in full. *The life of the mine workers,* they conclude, is not as bad as the union would have us believe. The mine patches are miserable places, but it's possible *choice and volition* explain it and not the low wages. It's possible the reason so many children work in the mines and mills is because they want to, not because wages are low. It's a settled fact that conditions are slowly improving. This industry is complicated and unique. So many factors conspire to limit production. Given that these *interruptions* are uniquely *incident to mining operations* and since this creates *uncertainty as to the number of days a miner* can actually work, the miners deserve some consideration. But only some. *The commission awards the miners an increase of 10 percent above wages as of April 1902.* All other union demands are rejected. The ruling reduces the working day for a small number of miners but not for the vast majority. The commission calls the miners' ton-wage basis too complicated to understand and refuses to abolish it. The coal companies are not compelled to recognize the union, says the commission, explaining that they have grave concerns about the United Mine Workers of America. We agree with Mitchell that the larger a labor union is, *the more businesslike and responsible it becomes.* But that doesn't describe the United Mine Workers. This is a union whose members destroy property, break contracts, and intimidate nonunion men by calling them scabs. This is a union that routinely violates the rights of management. They even give breaker boys a voice in union decisions. These are not the *most inviting inducements to entering into contractual relations.* Their ruling imposes a three-year contract set to begin on April 1, 1903. It includes the creation of a board of conciliation for the arbitration of disputes.

Union leaders and coal-company presidents celebrate the agreement. Mitchell predicts it *will result in great good and I am much pleased with it.* Darrow calls it a *good, substantial victory.* We didn't get everything, he says, but we got more than we had. *The finding itself is a practical recognition of the union.* The editor of the *United Mine Workers' Journal* agrees. The board of conciliation *means the recognition of the union is assured.* The Coxe Bros. attorney Simon Wolverton calls it *fair. The three-year agreement is an excellent one and will undoubtedly be satisfactory to all concerned.*

Most miners, however, come to a different conclusion. The Lehigh Coal and Navigation company refuses to pay the higher wage rate. Markle reclassifies muledrivers and cuts their pay. The first miners to file grievances under the new agreement are fired for filing grievances. Wildcat strikes sweep through the coalfields. Nearly two thousand Shamokin miners leave the mines after start times are arbitrarily changed. Twelve hundred walk off the job in Mahanoy City when muledrivers are forced to clock out before stabling the mules. The miners appeal to Mitchell for help, but he orders them back to the mines instead.

We have a contract, he tells them, and we mean to honor it. *While parts of the decision probably will not suit the miners*, he admits, at least it calls for the *withdrawal of the Coal and Iron Police, who are responsible for most of the trouble that occurs in the mining regions.* But this turns out to be only partly true. The arbitration commission concludes that the Coal and Iron Police should be disbanded, but only after it is replaced with public police. We must *have peace and order* in the coalfields, write the commissioners. The protection of property *should be maintained at any cost.* And this should be a cost borne by the state, and this can only be accomplished through the creation by legislation of *a regularly constituted constabulary.*

CONCLUSION

A WRECKING CREW

The history of the police can be found in the pleas for a state constabulary that were made by the anthracite coal-mine owners, which always grew loudest after a strike, like voices in an angry chorus. They cried for protection after the Long Strike of 1875, in their war against the Molly Maguires, even while their militias *patrolled the streets of Mauch Chunk with loaded rifles.* They pleaded for a new police and the *inauguration of a new order of things* after their *Committee of Vigilance and Safety* gunned down two striking miners in the streets of Scranton during the year of violence, 1877. *We could have routed* them all, they chanted, if only we had *a regular constabulary force* and not a temporary one. Even militia leaders joined the chorus after Homestead in 1892. *Citizen soldiers should not be called on to perform* strikebreaking work, concluded Isaac J. Wistar, general of the Pennsylvania militia, veteran of the Indian Wars, and president of the Pennsylvania Railroad. *The proper instrument would be a paid State constabulary.* There were calls for a better police after the sheriff's posse of merchants, mining foreman, and clerks from the coal companies murdered nineteen miners at Lattimer in 1897, a tragedy they chalked up to *our inefficient method of enforcing the law.* They called it a tragedy of law's absence, not its gunmen. The more they killed, the more cops they said they needed. *The sheriff, and even the deputies, were far less at fault than the statutes and the politicians and people who are responsible for the woeful defects in the statutes.*

The road to the institution of police was paved in the *mad days of riot* in the years leading up to the great anthracite strike of 1902, when the merchants and business interests first developed their own police and imposed their own order. Like the *Easton Greys* in 1877, who were sent in to *slaughter* the mine workers, and would have done it had the strikers not stopped them with *a shower of stones.* Or the armed *Citizen corps,* which patrolled the streets in support of the *Committees of Public Safety,* which seized the presses to keep the labor-friendly newspapers from stirring *up the mob elements.* Or the *Law and Order Brigade* that rode into Harrisburg in 1877 with *a whole car-load of ammunition,* courtesy of the *Philadelphia Railroad,* and broke *the backbone* of the strikers' *mob.* The Wilkes-Barre mine operators issued bonds to raise funds for the Scranton City Guard's arsenal, and then built it atop their mine. Every coal-carrying railroad offered the militia free trains for transportation. They built armories for the vigilantes and filled them with the newest guns. The Lackawanna Iron and Coal Co. donated land for rifle ranges. The Reading Railroad built spurs to militia encampments.

In the early years, the different militias and various city guards maintained informal affiliations. What started out as a loose federation of vigilance committees developed, strike by strike, into the Pennsylvania National Guard, *private police force of industry.* To the mine owners, it was never good enough, never large enough, never world-making enough. Always as much a problem as a solution—too slow to arrive, too full of undisciplined men—and always left them in the lurch after a strike. Its victories were only temporary and always came with *frightful consequences.* Instead of stable industrial production, it produced *hideous class hatreds* and lasting *enmity.* Even the militia leaders called for an alternative. We shouldn't be *aiding capital in its issues with labor,* concluded the Militia Bureau. Our strikebreaking produces low morale and makes it hard to recruit soldiers. The sacred duty of strikebreaking cannot be left to the militias and Pinkertons and sheriff's posses. The only practical solution was the *creation of a state constabulary.*

To make their case, the mine owners and industrialists developed a new language of order, a new vocabulary of threats and emergencies. A strike was not a strike, it was a riot and riots threaten industrial stability. A striker is a drunken idler. A parade is always a mob action. Freedom isn't found in labor, it's found in the wage. The police aren't just a body of armed strikebreakers, they're a promise of security. As long as police are part-time, the threat of combinations of labor will be full-time. They delivered their new arguments through a firehose of false promises. Only a state constabulary could *protect people outside of the cities against violent crimes.* Only a state constabulary could be stationed everywhere and *run down criminals wherever they may flee.* Only a state constabulary could be independent of the coal companies, insulated from vested interests and free from *party politics.* Everyone, even the working people, even the strikers, would benefit. Only a state constabulary could be tutored in the *just rights of labor, as well as property.* Only a state constabulary could replace the *powder and shot* of the militia with *less violent methods.* Only a state *constabulary could be called upon before any actual riot.* Only a state constabulary comprised of full-time, professional officers could be *trained for both preventive and repressive service.* Certainly the result will be *bruised heads,* but at least we won't have the *hideous corpses* left by the posse and militia.

They imagined a professional, democratic police and telescoped it into the past, where they discovered it to be heroic. *Had there been a small force of regularly organized State constabulary* at Lattimer in 1897, they claimed, *there would have been no bloodshed.* They pointed to the efficient violence of professional police as a reason for more police. And yet their pleas were always left unheeded. New Hampshire voters overwhelmingly rejected a state constabulary in the late 1860s. California tried and failed in 1880. When the Kansas governor John St. John proposed a state constabulary in 1882, the newspapers called him a *Czar* and his authoritarian ideas a *crazy fanaticism*. New York State tried and failed to pass a state constabulary law in the late 1890s. Time and time again, Pennsylvania voters refused to create a state constabulary, which many feared would be like a full-time version of the militias and sheriff's posses, and would exist only to patrol the coalfield as armed wings of the local boards of trade, sent by the bosses to *shoot down striking workmen in the name of the law.* Imagine a world with police like that, always on duty.

Find none of this in the official histories of the Pennsylvania State Police, which instead locates the origins of the police in the mind of Samuel Pennypacker, Republican governor of Pennsylvania, who was elected the same week the Jeddo miners were evicted from their homes and inaugurated the same week the Lattimer killers sang their praises to police at the Coal Strike Commission. Pennypacker, the police maker, promised *to replace the Coal and Iron Police* with a new state constabulary. He campaigned on it, said it would be his gift to the collieries, and was surprised when they told him they didn't want it. Why would we want a police force, the coal companies asked, that operated *independent of our orders?* When Pennypacker clarified that his proposal for a new, public police would not abolish private police, the bill became law. Most union leaders were unconcerned by Pennypacker's new police. The Pennsylvania Federation of Labor remained neutral during the debate, convinced that *no honorable man will join* the state police. After all, it would be small—225 cops spread over the entire state—and the bill describes it as a rural constabulary concerned more with the policing of hunters than the breaking up of strikes. Some progressives even supported the idea. *The Nation* magazine called the Pennsylvania State Police an *admirable model* that it hoped would be imitated by many other States. What could go wrong?

Pennypacker hired the wealthy Philadelphia liquor importer John C. Groome to create Pennsylvania's new state constabulary. Groome came recommended as someone who understood how strikebreaking had been done and how it could be done better. He served as captain of the First Troop Philadelphia City Cavalry, the oldest organized militia in the country. Its troopers, in Hussar hats and carrying glittering sabers, fought on blooded mounts in the Revolutionary War and in the War of 1812. They fought strikers at Homestead in 1892 and charged into Hazleton under Groome's command in 1897. Groome led the cavalry into Puerto Rico in 1898 and stood sentry while sheriffs' deputies carried out evictions in Hazleton in October and November of 1902. Groome knew the difference that a properly constituted state constabulary could make. It was one found not in weapons, tactics, training, or even in the character of the men who composed it, but in the power that came from taking the unlimited mandate of police to impose order and giving it a jurisdiction without limit, like a colonial occupation. Imagine the power of a force that could impose order through the use of violence under color of law wherever it was needed. Only police, whose discretion to impose order exceeds law, could effectively defend law.

He steamed to Dublin in September 1905 and spent three weeks with the Royal Irish Constabulary (RIC), touring its barracks and studying its *organization and practical workings*, learning how it managed the Land War evictions and how it suppressed the secret societies of the cities and countryside. He watched how it handled informants and quelled riots. When he returned from occupied Ireland, he declared that the Pennsylvania State Police *will be in every sense of the word military police and will be drilled and trained as a mounted force*. What good is a mandate to impose order that comes hamstrung by limits? He married war to police by recruiting *men accustomed to war and detectives' work*. He would outfit each trooper with a small pocket truncheon for hand-to-hand combat, a .38 Colt sidearm, a short-barreled .45 caliber Springfield rifle to be used in case of extreme disorder; and for crowd control, he issued each trooper a two-foot hickory club so dense it sank in water. He mounted his troopers on horses that met US cavalry standards and separated them into four commands billeted in four different barracks in two different coalfields. But what of the rural districts? No, Groome, said, when asked. *The farmers are pretty tame.* No need for any barracks in the rural areas. *The greatest need will be in the coal and iron regions*, he explained. Two troops occupied the western bituminous fields and two kept watch over the eastern anthracite coalfields. The mine workers called them *Pennypacker's Cossacks*, his *Black Hussars*. Mother Jones called them Irish Hessians and predicted *a brutal constabulary. It will soak these coalfields with the blood of men and of women.* Groome waved it all off. It's not like anyone can *tell a so-called striker from the tough or hired thug* anyway. A threat is a threat.

Order is what follows when the police become an occupation, as the Flying Squadron demonstrated. Groome's police were never not on duty. The Pennsylvania State Constabulary spent its first year conducting daily mounted patrols—a constant show of force—in twelve counties, suppressing the miners, arresting seventy-six strikers for rioting despite being *outnumbered by the lawless element*. The next year, owing to the *unsettled condition of affairs in the Anthracite Region of the State, caused by the suspension of work at all the Anthracite Coal Mines*, Groome *deemed advisable to patrol certain Sections of Schuylkill, Luzerne, and Carbon Counties*. If they loiter, they are a threat. His troopers marched into the *foreign colony near the Fernwood colliery* in 1906, where they chased Italian strikers from Mocanaqua *into the mountains*. If they run, they

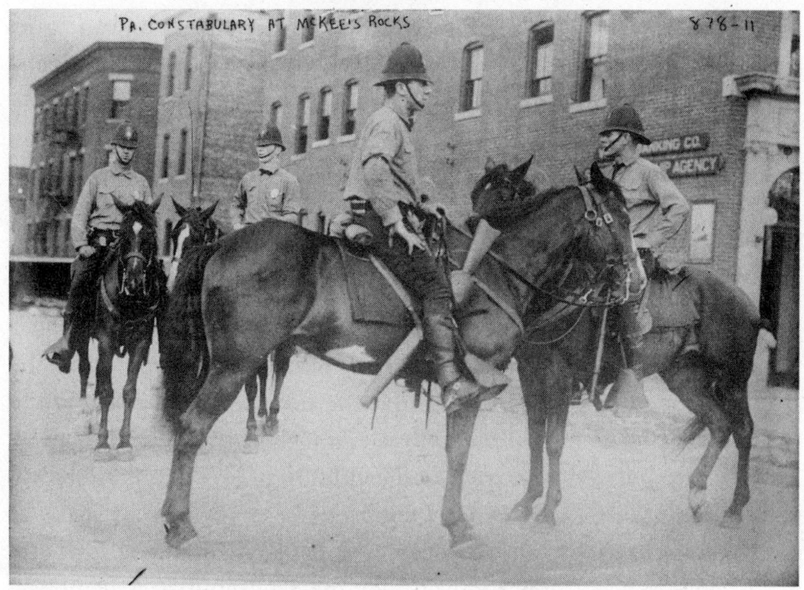

Troopers of the Pennsylvania State Constabulary. Courtesy: Library of Congress.

are a threat. His Troop B rode from Wyoming to the Franklin colliery near Wilkes-Barre where they *shackled* striking miners *in irons* and escorted scabs to and from work. Reporters asked if the state police had the authority to make such arrests. Yes, said a lieutenant, though we'd prefer to go *in and club the hell out of them.* Reporters heard rumors about a sergeant in Yatesville who reportedly told a crowd of people he'd *return and burn the place to the ground* if there were *any more disturbances.* Is it true? they asked Groome. Yes, he said. These are military men. They do what they're told.

With the state police now on patrol, the collieries had the unlimited jurisdiction their order required—the Coal and Iron Police, the sheriff's posse, the militia, and now the state constabulary. Every industry took advantage of Groome's new police. His troops rode into Chester in 1908 and broke the trolley workers' strike by guarding the constables while they ran the trolleys themselves. Undercover state cops infiltrated the strikers in the 1914 trolley strike in Hazleton and started fights with the scabs, inciting strikers to join them in the fray, arresting them when they did. Order had been brought to the coalfields, and the miners all agreed that conditions were *worse than in 1902*. Everything was being taken from the miners, *reduction by reduction*.

Like the smoke and soot released when coal is burned, the idea of a state constabulary took to the wind. In New York, the Chamber of Commerce *created a Committee for State Police* with offices on Wall Street. They wrote glossy reports on the terror of rural brigandage and the need for protection by the state police. *Life in the outlying and sparsely settled districts is nothing less than a continual condition of fear and peril for the inhabitants*, they wrote. They brought in Groome to speak at their meetings, and he described Pennsylvania as a formerly lawless place now safely under the pacifying heel of police. When the first efforts to create a state constabulary failed in New York, the businessmen hired Katherine Mayo, the political writer and so-called social reformer who would later defend colonialism in her 1927 book *Mother India*. Mayo, the *Mother of Police*, made propaganda films with Groome about how this new police would free us from the frightening *onslaught of rural crime* by *violent immigrants and blacks*. She illustrated the brochures she wrote about Groome with photos of his troops menacing striking mine workers. She testified before state commissions and gave talks to chambers of commerce. The campaign culminated in her 1917 book *Justice to All*, in which she lionized Groome and celebrated the Pennsylvania State Police. She filled it with anecdotes of manly troopers confronting *rioting mobs of foreigners* for whom *knives and guns are playthings*. She called attention to the laments of the unhappy famers and *intelligent English-speaking miner folk* in desperate need of protection from *hordes of savage Huns* and *mercurial* Italians and Poles.

The proponents of state police claimed the new police would protect working people. Mayo pointed to the 1902 strike as proof. *Whenever the miners elected to go out on strike. . . they invariably found the power of the State bought, paid for, and fighting as a partisan on their employers' side.* The state police replaced the *cruel and cowardly gunmen and riffraff* of the Coal and Iron Police, she wrote, with a *sober* and professional force. Teddy Roosevelt wrote the foreword. Finally, a friend to labor in the form of police. The evidence is clear, to oppose the state police now would be to side with *the lawless capitalists who used the law-defying Coal and Iron Police.* Who but *foolish or vicious labor leaders* would do that? Here it was again, as persistent as coal dust in a creek, the promise that the police will be a champion of labor, a protector of working people, as long as they took the wage they were given, respected management rights, and knew their place. New York created a state constabulary in 1917, the same year Groome got more pay and more cops for the Pennsylvania State Police. West Virginia followed in 1919, New Jersey in 1921, Delaware in 1923, Connecticut in 1924, Rhode Island in 1925. By 1941, the drifting smoke and soot of police had settled everywhere.

How did the Pennsylvania State Police protect working people? By beating them with clubs and infiltrating their unions and then placing them under constant surveillance. The state police sent undercover troopers on the trains to listen to the conversations of the miners during the strike of 1922. They loitered in the confectionery stores and cigar shops patroned by strikers, got haircuts in the barbershops where the Italians congregated, took note of threats overhead while playing nine-ball in upstairs pool halls. They forged union cards and smuggled themselves into union meetings. Their agents bought liquor for strikers in saloons and then wrote reports about *how much liquor is consumed* by the strikers. They spread rumors of *dynamite buried in the hills of East Millsboro and* then arrested the miners for burying explosives that no one ever found.

The state constabulary staked a claim to a new kind of police knowledge—an expertise conferred by a badge that conjured special knowledge of the strikers' secret plots to *give battle to the State Police and deputies at the first outbreak of trouble.* They filed reports that said every *man is armed* whether they were or not. They said the *foreigners are becoming restless,* turning *very radical,* which established that it was true. Their suggestions were given special attention. More guards should be hired, more private deputies must be brought on. The *loafers* and *young rowdies* congregating at the *B&O station* should be roughed up. *What is needed in this vicinity is a wrecking crew.*

The more the police became a special authority, the more threats emerged and the more emergencies the police declared. They patrolled the mine patches with mechanized squadrons of trucks mounted with large-caliber machine guns. The machine gun squadron from Troop E dug into the high ground above the Henderson mine during the 1922 bituminous strike *commanding a field of fire.* They fired their machine guns into the strikers' tent colony at night, terrifying the strikers and driving them away. They evicted strikers, set up checkpoints, conducted warrantless raids on homes and union locals, provided security on the trains that imported scabs, and arrested and held strike leaders without bail. Each troop included scout units and strikebreaking crews charged with protecting collieries and scabs. Each troop included intelligence units devoted to the infiltration of union locals. They embedded special agents with Pennsylvania National Guard cavalry troops. Wherever you found the wrecking crews of the police, you found starving miners on the roads *begging the farmers for food.*

The police occupation of the coalfields produced endless opportunities for the mine owners. They could now force the miners to work eleven-, twelve-, fourteen-hour days. Who would stop them? They reduced wages across the board and called it efficiency, celebrated it for its productivity. They saved money on mules by forcing the miners to push the three-ton coal cars from the headings to the face of the coal themselves. Plenty of cheap labor to replace the ones injured in the epidemic of ruptured backs and torn Achilles that followed. These were the lean years, in the 1920s, when the *weak-kneed workers* joined up with the foremen and *the espionage agents and the stool pigeons* in the proliferating company unions, like the Mutual Beneficial Association, which the Pennsylvania Railroad created to *break the solidarity of organized labor* in a campaign of terror and a *carnival of bloodshed.* Desperate miners passed local resolutions calling on the UMW to stand with the rank and file but found no support. The employers have *declared war upon the working class of this country.* Where are our leaders? We need a *nation-wide movement for a general strike of all labor.* It's either that, they told their national UMW organizers, or *stand condemned by the rank and file of labor as the allies of the employers.* John L. Lewis, Mitchell's replacement as president of the UMW, refused their pleas for help.

Schisms hardened into factions. Radical and militant groups splintered off. The National Miners Union, a communist-backed breakaway union, attracted the miners who despised Lewis's business-mindedness, who hated the way his district presidents acted like cops, ordering starving miners back to the mines. Some union leaders even started talking like cops. These militant miners, they complained, *swarmed into the coalfields* and brought *crime and disorder, violence and riot.* These dissidents fomented *hatred and hostility toward the existing order of things.* The UMW purged all those who challenged Lewis. Alexander Howat, the legendary coal miner from Kansas who spent years in and out of jail for challenging the law that made strikes, boycotts, pickets, and parades illegal, was driven from the UMW at its 1922 national convention in Indianapolis for challenging the conservative authority of Lewis. Only Mother Jones took to the convention floor to defend him. *If you fellows in Pennsylvania had kicked up the same kind of row* as Howat did in Kansas *when they saddled the mounted police on to you, we wouldn't have that established all over the country today.*

The Coal and Iron Police, assisted by the state police, *ran wild over western Pennsylvania, in 1927–28, cracking heads, terrorizing coal communities, entering miners' houses and tent colonies* in an endless campaign of arrests and shootings. This was the start of a new era, in which progressives condemned the bloodshed and lasting bitterness caused by police violence but called for more and more professional police as the solution. By the late 1920s the line between the state police and industrial police had so blurred that the rosters had become interchangeable. The state troopers, some of whom would later work as private deputies, and the private deputies, all of whom worked previously as state cops, occupied the mine patches around Coverdale in the strikes that swept through the bituminous fields in 1927–28. The striking miners, whom the mine owners called greedy, lived in cardboard shacks, and risked arrest just for fetching water from a well. The deputy sheriffs evicted them by tearing the roofs off their shanties. The union preached patience, but the desperate miners saw nothing worth being patient for.

In May 1935, a month before Pennsylvania would finally abolish the Coal and Iron Police, state troopers from the eastern anthracite coalfield's Wyoming Barracks launched an attack on the United Anthracite Miners of Pennsylvania, a breakaway mine-workers' union of nearly fifty thousand dues-paying members. Hundreds of cops with tape covering their badge numbers clubbed strikers on the street, and chased them into their homes, beating them in their kitchens. They hauled dozens of them to distant county jails, torturing them until they signed blank cards on which the police later typed the words *the treatment of police was good.* How many troopers were involved in the beatings, shootings, and arbitrary arrests? asked a civil rights commission that later investigated. Every one of them, said Thomas Maloney, president of the dissident union. *They're all in the same nest.* It's true, admitted Major Lynn G. Adams, Groome's replacement as superintendent of state police. *Some men had their heads busted. And I believe there will be some more.*

ACKNOWLEDGMENTS

I owe a great debt to the many librarians and archivists on whom I relied while researching this book, particularly Lucas Clawson at the Hagley Museum and Library, Harrison Wick at the Indiana University of Pennsylvania Special Collections and University Archive, John Fielding at the Anthracite Heritage Museum, Brett Reigh at the Pennsylvania State Archives, Anthony DiGiovanni at the Historical Society of Pennsylvania, Thomas White at the Duquesne University Archives and Special Collections, Hannah Kaufman at the Catholic University of America Archives, and the many archivists at the National Archives and Records Administration in College Park, Maryland. A Henry Belin du Pont Research Fellowship from the Hagley Museum and Library gave me a month in their amazing Soda House archive. Many thanks to Roger Horowitz and Carol Lockman. Financial support from the University of New Mexico Research Allocations Committee and the Department of American Studies covered the costs of multiple trips to many archives.

I worked out some of the ideas that appear in this book in formal and informal talks I gave over the past few years. Thanks to John Beck at Michigan State University and his Our Daily Work/Our Daily Lives speaker series. Greg Hargreaves and the participants in the Hagley lecture series offered terrific questions and thoughtful suggestions that improved this book. My University of New Mexico colleagues, Jennifer Denetdale,

Alyosha Goldstein, Rebecca Schreiber, Katie Holscher, and Frank Galarte heard me present parts of the book. I'm grateful for their attention, insights, and critical suggestions. I've talked at length about this book to many people, particularly Andy Doolen, Lorena Oropeza, Tyler Wall, John Hintz, Ernesto Longa, Roger Horowitz, and Bill Bradley. This book is better for their feedback, enthusiasm, and support. I benefited from the bottomless generosity of John and Michelle Hintz, who opened their home to me on my many trips to eastern Pennsylvania. This book was made so much better by Trevor Perri's copyediting, John Hintz's great map, and the terrific editorial work and guidance of Anthony Arnove, Jameka Williams, Eric Kerl, and Rory Fanning at Haymarket Books.

Toni Kuehn and our daughters, Willa and Harper, watched this book consume me over the course of the past two years. The only thing I've loved more than that is the three of them.

REFERENCES

NOTES FOR PAGES 1 TO 4

Introduction: Dig Another Grave

the effigy of a cop's *corpse*: "Judge Musmanno as Orator Accidentally Hurt by Brick," *Pittsburgh Post-Gazette*, June 17, 1935, p. 5; "Musmanno Hit by Brick as Miners Celebrate in Waynesburg," *Pittsburgh Sun-Telegraph*, June 16, 1935, p. 2.

whose *bill killed the system*: Ray Sprigle, "Murder in the Police Barracks, The John Borcoski Story," *Pittsburgh Post-Gazette*, April 24, 1949.

***we will dig another grave*:** "Judge Musmanno as Orator Accidentally Hurt by Brick."

whiskey from a pint that Watts pulled from his coat: Testimony of Patsy Caruso, Michael Musmanno Collection, Coal and Iron Police Sub-group, Series III: Borcoski Case, Box 3, Folder 4: Testimonies, Duquesne University Archives, Pittsburgh, PA.

John Borcoski: Newspapers and archives used multiple spellings of his last name, which included Barcoski, Barkoski, Borckovski, and Barkowski. I've chosen to use Borcoski throughout the text as this is the most common spelling found in the Michael Musmanno Collection.

The only man *who'd smoke a Lucky is a klansman*: Testimony of Corporal O. J. Mechling, Michael Musmanno Collection, Coal and Iron Police Sub-group, Series III: Borcoski Case, Box 3, Folder 4: Testimonies, Duquesne University Archives, Pittsburgh, PA.

Watts chased after Borcoski: "History of the Borcoski Case," n.d., Michael Musmanno Collection, Coal and Iron Police Sub-group, Series III: Borcoski Case, Box 3, Folder 1, Duquesne University Archives, Pittsburgh, PA; "Dollar or Daughter, Rule of Coal Cops, Widow Says," *Pittsburgh Post-Gazette*, February 13, 1929.

***It was none of my business*:** Scrapbook 2, Michael Musmanno Collection, Coal and Iron Police Sub-group, Series III: Borcoski Case, Box 3, Folder 35: Coal & Iron Controversy, Duquesne University Archives, Pittsburgh, PA.

but not out of any concern for Borcoski or Higgins: "Claim Cutting Charge 'Frame Up' By Police," *Pittsburgh Post-Gazette*, February 13, 1929, p. 4.

When I arrived, Patterson would say: Testimony of Dr. J. M. Patterson, Michael Musmanno Collection, Coal and Iron Police Sub-group, Series III: Borcoski Case, Box 3, Folder 4: Testimonies, Duquesne, University Archives, Pittsburgh, PA.

I feel like having a workout: "Bereaved," Michael Musmanno Collection, Coal and Iron Police Sub-group, Series III: Borcoski Case, Box 3, Folder 8: *The Bulletin Index: Pittsburgh's Weekly Newsmagazine*, Duquesne University Archives, Pittsburgh, PA.

I saw him kick Borcoski violently in the side: Testimony of Corporal O. J. Mechling.

until he heard the sound of bones breaking: Scrapbook 1, February 1929, Michael Musmanno Collection, Coal and Iron Police Sub-group, Series III: Borcoski Case, Box 3, Folder 34: Coal & Iron Police Controversy, Duquesne University Archives, Pittsburgh, PA.

delighting in the impact of the whip, club and fist upon bare flesh: "The System at Fault," n.d., Michael Musmanno Collection, Coal and Iron Police Sub-group, Series III Borkowski Case, Box 3, Folder 9: Newspaper Clippings, Duquesne University Archives, Pittsburgh, PA.

he heard ribs snap from the other room: Scrapbook 1, February 1929, Michael Musmanno Collection, Coal and Iron Police Sub-group, Series III: Borcoski Case, Box 3, Folder 34: Coal & Iron Police Controversy, Duquesne University Archives, Pittsburgh, PA.

I was afraid of them: Scrapbook 2, Michael Musmanno Collection, Coal and Iron Police Sub-group, Series III: Borcoski Case, Box 3, Folder 35: Coal & Iron Controversy, Duquesne University Archives, Pittsburgh, PA.

His *rib structure was fractured*: Testimony of Higgins, "History of the Barcoski Case," n.d., Michael Musmanno Collection, Coal and Iron Police Sub-group, Series III: Borcoski Case, Box 3, Folder 1, Duquesne University Archives, Pittsburgh, PA.

What did you do with my husband?: "Dollar or Daughter, Rule of Coal Cops, Widow Says."

life isn't safe: "Dollar or Daughter, Rule of Coal Cops, Widow Says."

Watts had murdered a Black man named M. C. Watkins: "Cop Pardoned in Death Case," *Pittsburgh Post-Gazette*, February 13, 1929.

without moral stamina: Sprigle, "Murder in the Police Barracks: The John Borcoski Story."

Watts and Lyster were convicted: "Bereaved"; "The Battle is Not Won," Michael Musmanno Collection, Coal and Iron Police Sub-group, Series

III: Borcoski Case, Box 3, Folder 9: Newspaper Clippings, Duquesne University Archives, Pittsburgh, PA.

calling Lyster a fine officer: "Estimate of Lyster Given by Coal Head," *Pittsburgh Post-Gazette*, February 13, 1929.

won a $13,000 settlement . . . and lost it to the bank a year later: "Bereaved."

The 1865 statute that created the Coal and Iron Police: 1865, P.L. 225, amended 1866, P.L. 1866.

but their powers are more general: See Bunting v. P.A. R.R., Co., 284 Pa. 117, 120; Finefrock v. North Cent. Ry Co., 58 Pa. Super. 52, 59; Naugle v. P.R.R. Co., 83 Pa. Super. 528.

Wherever you found a laboring poor: See Sidney L. Harring, *Policing a Class Society: The Experience of American Cities, 1865–1915* (Rutgers: Rutgers University Press, 1983); William T. Martin, "Industrial Police Stir Pennsylvania," *New York Times*, February 1, 1931.

revealed the power of a unified working class: Harring, *Policing a Class Society*, 106.

some like the old slave patrols: See Philip L. Reichel, "Southern Slave Patrols as a Transitional Police Type," *American Journal of Police* 7 (1988): 51; James Loewen, *Sundown Towns: A Hidden Dimension of American Racism* (New York: The New Press, 2005).

Railroad police operated in North Carolina, Rhode Island, and North Dakota: Letter from Dennis Brummitt, AG of C to Musmanno, October 22, 1930; Letter from Benjamin M. McLyman, AG of Rhode Island to Musmanno, October 21, 1930; Letter from Harold Shaft, Assistant AG of ND to Musmanno, October 23, 1930, Michael Musmanno Collection, Coal and Iron Police Sub-group; Series I: Legislation Attempting to Outlaw Coal and Iron Police, Box 2, Folder 13: Correspondence, Duquesne University Archives, Pittsburgh, PA.

West Virginia and Kentucky allowed collieries: Letter from James W. Cammack, AG of Kentucky to Musmanno, October 24, 1930; Letter from Howard B. Lee, AG of WV to Musmanno, October 22, 1930, Michael Musmanno Collection, Coal and Iron Police Sub-group; Series I: Legislation Attempting to Outlaw Coal and Iron Police, Box 2, Folder 13: Correspondence, Duquesne University Archives, Pittsburgh, PA.

California, New York, and Rhode Island: Letter from Benjamin M. McLyman; Letter from the Office of Hamilton Ward, AG of NY to Musmanno, October 25, 1930; Letter from the office of U. S. Webb, AG of CA to Musmanno, October 27, 1930, Michael Musmanno Collection, Coal and Iron Police Sub-group; Series I: Legislation Attempting to Outlaw Coal and Iron Police, Box 2, Folder 13: Correspondence, Duquesne University Archives, Pittsburgh, PA.

Virginia, South Carolina, Iowa, South Dakota, and Minnesota: Letter from Jno. R. Saunders, AG of Virginia, October 21, 1930; Letter from John Fletcher, AG of Iowa to Musmanno, October 22, 1930; Letter from M. Q. Sharpe, AG of SD to Musmanno, October 22, 1930; Letter from William H. Gurnee, Assistant AG of Minnesota to Musmanno, October 23, 1930; Letter from John M. Daniel, AG of SC to Musmanno, October 31, 1930, Michael Musmanno Collection, Coal and Iron Police Sub-group; Series I: Legislation Attempting to Outlaw Coal and Iron Police, Box 2, Folder 13: Correspondence, Duquesne University Archives, Pittsburgh, PA.

***under certain contingencies or extraordinary circumstances*:** Letter from E. C. Shively, First Assistant Attorney General, Ohio to Michael Musmanno, October 24, 1930; Letter from Helen Kelley, Secretary to the Connecticut AG to Musmanno, October 25, 1930; Letter from Geo. M. Napier, AG of Georgia to Musmanno, October 22, 1930; Letter from Charlie C. McCall, AG of Alabama to Musmanno, October 23, 1930, Michael Musmanno Collection, Coal and Iron Police Sub-group; Series I: Legislation Attempting to Outlaw Coal and Iron Police, Box 2, Folder 13: Correspondence, Duquesne University Archives, Pittsburgh, PA.

***Illinois prohibited so-called industrial police*:** Letter from Oscar E. Carlstrom, AG of IL to Musmanno, October 23, 1930, Michael Musmanno Collection, Coal and Iron Police Sub-group; Series I: Legislation Attempting to Outlaw Coal and Iron Police, Box 2, Folder 13: Correspondence, Duquesne University Archives, Pittsburgh, PA.

Maine, Indiana, and Washington let cities outsource policing: Letter from Clement F. Robinson, AG of Maine to Musmanno, October 23, 1930; Letter from Merle Wall, Deputy AG, Indiana (Law Enforcement) to Musmanno, October 24, 1930; Letter from John H. Dunbar, AG of Washington to Musmanno, October 27, 1930, Michael Musmanno Collection, Coal and Iron Police Sub-group; Series I: Legislation Attempting to Outlaw Coal and Iron Police, Box 2, Folder 13: Correspondence, Duquesne University Archives, Pittsburgh, PA.

every home and hearth up and down the Eastern Seaboard: Robert J. Cornell, *The Anthracite Coal Strike of 1902* (New York: Russell & Russell, 1971), 8.

a matter of national security: Robley D. Evans, "Reserve our Anthracite for our Navy," *The North American Review*, vol. 184 (1907): 246.

Business professors claimed it kickstarted the iron industry: Alfred D. Chandler, "Anthracite Coal and the Beginnings of the

Industrial Revolution in the United States," *Business History Review* 46, no. 2 (1972): 141–81.

tear gas, buckshot and machine guns: Gifford Pinchot, "Foreword," in *Report to Governor Gifford Pinchot*, ed. Commission on Special Policing in Industry, Department of Labor and Industry, Commonwealth of Pennsylvania, Special Bulletin, No. 38, October 9, 1934.

Private cops put sixty bullets in one striker's leg: Gates School, August 10, 1934, Michael Musmanno Collection, Coal and Iron Police Sub-group Series III: Borcoski Case Box 3, Folder 37: List of Incidents Involving Coal and Iron Police, Duquesne University Archives, Pittsburgh, PA.

They have been guilty of every crime on the calendar: Musmanno Speeches, Michael Musmanno Collection, Coal and Iron Police Sub-group, Series III: Borcoski Case, Box 2, Folder 1, Duquesne University Archives, Pittsburgh, PA.

the sovereignty of the Commonwealth: Musmanno, "Funeral Oration," Michael Musmanno Collection, Coal and Iron Police Sub-group, Series I: "Legislation Attempting to Outlaw Coal and Iron Police," Box 2, Folder 7, Duquesne, University Archives, Pittsburgh, PA.

and everything that divided them: On the role race and ethnicity play in class formation, and, specifically, the way bosses and white wage laborers divide workers by race and ethnicity, see David Roediger, *The Wages of Whiteness: Race and the Making of the American Working Class* (New York: Verso Books, 2022).

We have the state constabulary law: Letter from Lucius Robinson to Adrian Iselin, Jr., October 20, 1910, Collection 51: Rochester and Pittsburgh Coal & Iron Company, Executive Correspondence, 1909–1910, Box 2c, Folder 10: LWR 1910, October 20–28, Special Collections and University Archive, Indiana University of Pennsylvania, Indiana, PA.

a fight Samuel Gompers called the most important single incident in the labor movement: Samuel Gompers, *Seventy Years of Life and Labor: An Autobiography*, vol. 2 (New York: E. P. Dutton & Co., 1925), 126; Mitchell's quote appears in a letter he wrote to Mother Jones, May 10, 1902, reprinted in Cornell, *The Anthracite Coal Strike of 1902*, 91.

Chapter 1: A Good Practical Miner

rich deposits of a coastal plain's bogs and rias gone into hiding: For a survey of carboniferous fossil plants in the anthracite coal basin, see John Okeskyshyn, *Fossil Plants from the Anthracite Coalfields of Eastern Pennsylvania*, General Geology Report 72 (Harrisburg: Department of Environmental Resources, 1988).

shafts that drop from the surface like elevators: For a description of the different types of mine openings, see Harold W. Aurand, *Coalcracker Culture: Work and Values in Pennsylvania Anthracite, 1835–1935* (Selinsgrove: Susquehanna University Press, 2003).

gangways and muleways that lead to where the miners work: Aurand, *Coalcracker Culture*, 45–52.

the black damp is weak: Testimony of James Gallagher, Transcript of the Anthracite Coal Strike Commission, December 6, 1902, Scranton, PA, Vol. 13, Box 3, p. 1663.

***butty*:** When working under a contract, the term *butty* referred to a miner's partner.

Some pitch nearly perpendicular to the surface: For a description of the pitch and run of the veins, see "Highland No. 5–Gamma Vein Plane L," Jeddo Highland Coal Co. Records, MG 497, Box 3, Folder 116, Anthracite Heritage Museum, Scranton, PA; Testimony of John Veith, Mining Superintendent for Philadelphia & Reading Coal & Iron Co., Transcript of the Anthracite Coal Strike Commission, January 29, 1903, Philadelphia, PA, NARA II, Vol. 46, Box 7, pp. 7820–81.

There is no standard rule or guide: Wickeizer: "There are no two places alike. I find when I go to a new place it is different." Q: "How long does it take you to acquire that special experience?" Wickeizer: "Just as soon as I fire a couple of blasts.": Testimony of J. P. Wickeizer, Contract Miner at People's Coal Co.'s Oxford Colliery, Transcript of the Anthracite Coal Strike Commission, January 24, 1903, Philadelphia, PA, NARA II, Vol. 42, Box 7, p. 7187.

***It is a piece of work that can never be learned*:** Testimony of William H. Dettrey, Transcript of the Anthracite Coal Strike Commission, December 3, 1902, Scranton, PA, NARA II, Vol. 10, Box 2, p. 1172.

***water gushes out of them*:** Testimony of P. D. Gallagher, Transcript of the Anthracite Coal Strike Commission, December 9, 1902, Scranton, PA, NARA II, Vol. 15, Box 3, p. 1881.

Some holes fill the breast with pockets of methane: Testimony of William H. Dettrey, pp. 1165–66.

***but an inexperienced man loses powder there*:** Testimony of David F. Evans, Transcript of the Anthracite Coal Strike Commission, January 23, 1903, Philadelphia, PA, NARA II, Vol. 41, Box 6, p. 6938.

***I went to pull the pin out*:** Testimony of John Price, Transcript of the Anthracite Coal Strike Commission, December 5, 1902, Scranton, PA, NARA II, Vol. 12, Box 2, p. 1546.

bobtail check: Aurand, *Coalcracker Culture*, 92.

***A man may go to look after his fuse*:** Testimony of Gibbons, Transcript of the Anthracite Coal Strike Commission, November 21, 1902, Scranton, PA, NARA, Vol. 8, Box 2, p. 972.

***I squeezed the fuse to squeeze the dead fire out*:** Testimony of David J. Davis, Transcript of the Anthracite Coal Strike Commission, December 5, 1902, Scranton, PA, NARA II, Vol. 12, Box 2, p. 1548.

***I told the boss one day, I says*:** Testimony of Neal McDonigle, Transcript of the Anthracite Coal Strike Commission, December 9, 1902, Scranton, PA. NARA II, Vol. 15, Box 3, p. 1872.

***weigh it on scales by the pound*:** See "The Hard Working Miner," in *Minstrels of the Mine Patch: Songs and Stories of the Anthracite Industry*, edited by George Korson (Hatboro: Folklore Associates, 1964), 226–27.

***It is something so thick you cannot go through*:** Testimony of Frank Ray, Transcript of the Anthracite Coal Strike Commission, December 6, 1902, Scranton, PA, NARA II, Vol. 13, Box 3, p. 1685.

pockmarks: For a description of the pockmarked face of anthracite coal, see James C. Hower, Susan M. Rimmer, Maria Mastalerz, and Nicola J. Wagner, "Notes on the Mechanisms of Coal Metamorphism in the Pennsylvania Anthracite Fields," *International Journal of Coal Geology* 202 (2019): 161–70.

sounding the top coal: See M. Accursia, "Polish Miners in Luzerne County," *Polish American Studies* 3, no. 1/2 (1946): 11.

***are always getting larger*:** Testimony of James Gallagher, Transcript of the Anthracite Coal Strike Commission, December 8, 1902, Scranton, PA, NARA II, Vol. 14, Box 3, p. 1720.

***the coal in a manner that permitted a maximum amount of space*:** Aurand, *Coalcracker Culture*, 88.

***a shell of slate covering coal*:** Testimony of Paul Dunleavy, Transcript of the Anthracite Coal Strike Commission, December 8, 1902, Scranton, PA, NARA II, Vol. 14, Box 3, p. 1766.

***No matter how heavy we loaded our cars*:** Testimony of Paul Dunleavy, p. 1762.

***a half or maybe three-quarters of what you deliver*:** Testimony of Mike Midlick, Transcript of the Anthracite Coal Strike Commission, December 3, 1902, Scranton, PA, NARA II, Vol. 10, Box 2, p. 1186.

bosses make their money by mining you: Aurand, *Coalcracker Culture*, 107–14.

It's a magical thing—a rock that burns: See Gary E. Stinchcomb, R. Michael Stewart, Timothy C. Messner, Lee C. Nordt, Steven G. Driese, Peter M. Allen, "Using Event Stratigraphy to Map the Anthropocene—An Example from the Historic Coal Mining Region in Eastern Pennsylvania, USA," *Anthropocene* 2 (2013): 42–50.

Look at this new working class it made: See Alfred Chandler, "Anthracite Coal and the Beginnings of the Industrial Revolution in the United States," *The Business History Review* 46, no. 2 (1972): 141–81.

They order you to load five cars but won't even give you four: Testimony of John A. Davis, Certified Miner at D, L & W's Brisbin Colliery, Transcript of the Anthracite Coal Strike Commission, February 4, 1903, Philadelphia, PA, NARA II, Vol. 50, Box 9, p. 8848.

Watch it sink in water: Testimony of Dr. W. M. L. Coplin, Transcript of the Anthracite Coal Strike Commission, February 5, 1903, Philadelphia, PA, NARA II, Vol. 51, Box 9, p. 9057.

refugees from villages along the Dalmatian coast: See Emily Greene Balch, *Our Slavic Fellow Citizens* (New York: Charities Publication Committee, 1910), 37; Victor R. Greene, *The Slavic Community on Strike: Immigrant Labor in Pennsylvania Anthracite* (Notre Dame: University of Notre Dame Press, 1968).

***so narrow they had to walk on their neighbor's land*:** Balch, *Our Slavic Fellow Citizens*, 40.

They were recruited here: "The Slavs themselves say that there was an effort made, especially by the individual operator, to import cheap labor into the anthracite coalfield. It was done by the operators using ship agents, and getting men in New York to watch the vessels coming in and to turn the tide of Slav immigration into the coalfields": See Testimony of Rev. Peter Roberts, Transcript of the Anthracite Coal Strike Commission, 19 November 1902, Scranton, PA, NARA II, Vol. 6, Box 1, p. 759.

***We want mainly good Italians, Polanders and Hungarians*:** Letter from Lucius Robinson to A. J. Davis, July 11, 1902, Collection 51: R&P Coal and Iron Co., Box 1, Folder 7, Early Executive Correspondence Letter Book, 1902. Indiana University of Pennsylvania, Special Collections and University Archive.

They had their mine foremen pay immigrant breaker boys: Testimony of Andrew Matty, Transcript of the Anthracite Coal Strike Commission, December 4, 1902, Scranton, PA, NARA II, Vol. 11, Box 2, pp. 1236–27.

***We would like to get green labor mostly*:** Letter from Lucius Robinson to A. J. Davis, July 11, 1902; Letter from Lucius Robinson to All Superintendents, July 21, 1902, Collection 51: R&P Coal and Iron Co., Box 1, Folder 7, Early

Executive Correspondence Letter Book, 1902. Indiana University of Pennsylvania, Special Collections and University Archive.

ticket peddlers set up podiums in market towns: Mark Wyman, *Round-Trip to America: The Immigrants Return to Europe, 1880–1930* (Ithaca: Cornell University Press, 1993), 25.

***See if there is still justice in the world*:** Balch, *Our Slavic Fellow Citizens*, 52.

Don't stand out: Balch, *Our Slavic Fellow Citizens*, 350.

found the man from the photo waiting for them: Greene, *The Slavic Community on Strike*, 40.

No matter where they came from, the newspapers called them: Testimony of David F. Evans, 6942; Alexander Trachtenberg, *The History of Legislation for the Protection of Coal Miners in Pennsylvania, 1824–1915* (New York: International Publisher, 1943), 105–51.

***it ain't law they think about, it's money*:** Balch, *Our Slavic Fellow Citizens*, 368.

Their wages were swallowed by deductions: Aurand, *Coalcracker Culture*, 92; Testimony of T. Edward Ross, Transcript of the Anthracite Coal Strike Commission, January 27, 1903, Philadelphia, PA, NARA II, Vol. 44, Box 7, pp. 7409–59.

Saloons on every block because each served as a kind of community center: Greene, *The Slavic Community on Strike*, 48.

Hazleton miners sent fifty thousand dollars a month to Europe: Greene, *The Slavic Community on Strike*, 174.

the Slavish *are more lawless than the other miners*: Testimony of John Mitchell, Pres. of UMWA, Transcript of the Anthracite Coal Strike Commission, November 14, 1902, Scranton, PA, NARA II, Vol. 2, Box 1, p. 103.

***We cannot talk with these people*:** Testimony of John Veith, Mining Superintendent for Philadelphia & Reading Coal & Iron Co., Transcript of the Anthracite Coal Strike Commission, January 29, 1903, Philadelphia, PA, NARA II, Vol. 46, Box 7, p. 7909.

***desirable emigrants who could be induced to go into the mines*:** Letter from the General Manager to All Superintendents, July 23, 1902, Collection 51: R&P Coal and Iron Co., Box 1, Folder 7, Early Executive Correspondence Letter Book, 1902, Special Collections and University Archive, Indiana University of Pennsylvania, Indiana, PA.

***to be strikers and cast-off labor from other mines*:** Letter from the General Manager to A. J. Davis, Agt., July 11, 1902, Collection 51: R&P Coal and Iron Co., Box 1, Folder 7, Early Executive Correspondence Letter Book,

1902, Special Collections and University Archive, Indiana University of Pennsylvania, Indiana, PA.

pay us $2.38 instead: Peter Roberts, *Anthracite Coal Communities: A Study of the Demography, the Social, Educational and Moral Life of the Anthracite Region* (New York: Macmillan, 1904), 39.

***their heavy fists*:** Accursia, "Polish Miners in Luzerne County," 7.

the Slavic miners launched their own work stoppages: Roberts, *Anthracite Coal Communities*, 39; "Strikers on the Rampage," *New York Times*, August 10, 1887; "Strikers Rioting Again," *New York Times*, February 5, 1888.

Polish and Italian women organized huge marches and parades in the streets: "The Coal Operators Are Becoming More Cheerful," *Miners' Journal*, May 27, 1902; "Women Drove off Deputies," *Miners' Journal*, June 3, 1902; "They Return." *Miners' Journal*, June 4, 1902; "Heavy Rains are Flooding the Anthracite Coal Mines," *Miners' Journal*, July 4, 1902; see also Grace Palladino, *Another Civil War: Labor, Capital, and the State in the Anthracite Regions of Pennsylvania, 1840–68* (Champaign: University of Illinois Press, 1990), 99; Greene, *The Slavic Community on Strike*, 143; Aurand, *Coalcracker Culture*, 125; on social and economic status and the ways women navigated gender, ethnic, and class identities and divides, see Victoria C. Westmont, "Creating Anthracite Women: The Roles of Architecture and Material Culture in Identity Formation in Pennsylvania Anthracite Company Towns, 1854–1940" (PhD diss., University of Maryland, 2019); Emma L. Staffaroni, "'What Could You Do with a Dollar?' An Italian-American Woman's Breadwinning and Autonomy in Coal Country, Pennsylvania, 1929–1941" (MA thesis, Sarah Lawrence College, 2013); Balch, *Our Fellow Slavic Citizens*.

joined with the Slavs instead: Greene, *Our Slavic Fellow Citizens*, xv.

saloon in the house of a woman widowed in the last mine disaster: See George Korson, *Minstrels of the Mine Patch: Songs and Stories of the Anthracite Industry* (State College: Pennsylvania State University Press, 2016), 3; For an explanation of the survival strategies of widows, see statement of Clarence Darrow, Transcript of the Anthracite Coal Strike Commission, January 24, 1903, Philadelphia, PA, NARA II, Vol. 42, Box 7, p. 7136.

***It is a long time since I know'd in Jeddo*:** Testimony of James Gallagher, Transcript of the Anthracite Coal Strike Commission, February 5, 1903, Philadelphia, PA, NARA II, Vol. 51, Box 9, p. 9008.

***You can put an eleven-foot plank inside the car now*:** Testimony of James Gallagher, Transcript of the Anthracite Coal Strike Commission, February 5, 1903, p. 9010.

unless a man is half-killed, he is not hurt: Testimony of James Gallagher, Transcript of the Anthracite Coal Strike Commission, December 6, 1902, pp. 1636.

How many times you get half killed?: Testimony of James Gallagher, Transcript of the Anthracite Coal Strike Commission, December 6, 1902, pp. 1636, 1640.

Every evening we were not able to get out of the mines: Testimony of Andrew Hannik, Transcript of the Anthracite Coal Strike Commission, December 9, 1902, Philadelphia, PA, NARA II, Vol. 15, Box 3, p. 1891.

I was working four-handed with Henry Coll: Testimony of James Gallagher, Transcript of the Anthracite Coal Strike Commission, December 6, 1902, p. 1636.

a *man by the name of Kennedy*: Testimony of James Gallagher, Transcript of the Anthracite Coal Strike Commission, December 6, 1902, p. 1637.

I lay there unconscious for a good while: Testimony of James Gallagher, Transcript of the Anthracite Coal Strike Commission, December 6, 1902, p. 1637.

Henry *had his feet the way I have mine against the chair here*: Testimony of James Gallagher, Transcript of the Anthracite Coal Strike Commission, December 6, 1902, pp. 1,637–38.

Of course, the other story is more simpler to tell: Testimony of James Gallagher, Transcript of the Anthracite Coal Strike Commission, December 6, 1902, pp. 1638–39.

I got one that nearly finished me: Testimony of Henry Coll, Transcript of the Anthracite Coal Strike Commission, December 9, 1902, Scranton, PA, NARA II, Vol. 15, Box 3, p. 1899.

A piece of coal hit me in the eye: Testimony of Henry Coll, Transcript of the Anthracite Coal Strike Commission, December 9, 1902, pp. 1902.

a glass eye: Testimony of Henry Coll, Transcript of the Anthracite Coal Strike Commission, December 9, 1902, p. 1,899.

support the parents in idleness: Statement of William Taylor, St. Clair Coal Company lawyer, Transcript of the Anthracite Coal Strike Commission, January 29, 1902, Philadelphia, PA, NARA II, Vol. 46, Box 7, pp. 7881.

I never seen him until when a man got his leg or arm broke or crushed up: Testimony of James Gallagher, Transcript of the Anthracite Coal Strike Commission, December 8, 1902, pp. 1712.

I'm the fella from the mine that day: Testimony of James Gallagher, Transcript of the Anthracite Coal Strike Commission, December 8, 1902, p. 1713.

***I said, I pronounce that man committed suicide*:** Testimony of Edward Roderick, Transcript of the Anthracite Coal Strike Commission, December 17, 1902, Scranton, PA, NARA II, Vol. 22, Box 3, p. 3203; Testimony of James Gallagher, Transcript of the Anthracite Coal Strike Commission, December 8, 1902, p. 1714.

***Why did you do that?*:** Testimony of James Gallagher, Transcript of the Anthracite Coal Strike Commission, December 8, 1902, pp. 1713–14.

***On account of the man was not qualified to work*:** Testimony of Edward Roderick, Transcript of the Anthracite Coal Strike Commission, December 17, 1902, p. 3213.

***A great many of them are due to carelessness and misjudgment*:** Testimony of James Gallagher, Transcript of the Anthracite Coal Strike Commission, December 8, 1902, pp. 1,725; Testimony of Edward Roderick, Transcript of the Anthracite Coal Strike Commission, December 17, 1902, p. 3236.

***You mean to say that men who work a dangerous place*:** Excerpt of Clarence Darrow, Lawyer for the United Mine Workers, cross-examining Edward Roderick, Mine Inspector, 1st Anthracite District, Transcript of the Anthracite Coal Strike Commission, December 17, 1902, Scranton, PA, NARA II, Vol. 22, Box 3, pp. 3229–36.

into the bottom of the Susquehanna River: See Robert P. Wolensky, Kenneth C. Wolensky, and Nicole H. Wolensky, *Voices of the Knox Mine Disaster: Stories, Remembrances, and Reflections of the Anthracite Coal Industry's Last Major Catastrophe, January 22, 1959* (Harrisburg, PA: Pennsylvania Historical and Museum Commission, 2005).

leaving the dragged-out corpses: Aurand, *Coalcracker Culture*, 97–98.

factories that sometimes blow up: "Blown to Death: Ten Girls Meet a Sad Fate," *Wilkes-Barre Sunday Leader*, March 3, 1889, 7.

An old man carrying a bucket full of coal: Frank Norris, "Life in the Mining: A Study in Strike-Time of the Conditions of Living in Representative Mining Towns," *Everybody's Magazine*, September 1902, p. 246.

scanning for the Coal and Iron Police: Testimony of Frank Hatcher, Coal & Iron Police Lieutenant for the Henry Clay Colliery, Transcript of the Anthracite Coal Strike Commission, January 30, 1903, Philadelphia, PA, NARA II, Vol. 47, Box 8, p. 8127.

By thirty years old, in 1899, he was the president of the United Mine Workers of America: See Craig Phelan, *Divided Loyalties: The Public and Private Life of Labor Leader John Mitchell* (New York: SUNY Press, 1994).

1901 was the year 150,000 miners: "About 35% of the total production in the years past has gone into the washeries, or what are now the washeries—the culm banks": Testimony of W. W. Ruley, Coal Production Statistitican, Transcript of the Anthracite Coal Strike Commission, February 2, 1903, Philadelphia, PA, NARA II, Vol. 48, Box 8, p. 8255. The total amount removed from the ground in 1901 would include coal and all culm, which would bring the total close to 100 million tons, or about 140 million cubic yards. The anthracite coalfields comprise a 490-square-mile area, or 294,400 acres, which means that 140 million cubic yards would cover the entire region in dirt 177 feet deep. On water: "During the decade between 1902 and 1912, for example, the industry pumped an average of one billion tons of water to the surface annually." Aurand, *Coalcracker Culture*, 56. It would take 95,875,000 gallons of water to flood the coalfields one foot deep. One billion tons of water, or one trillion gallons, would flood the entire anthracite region 10,000 feet deep.

so their families could afford food: Testimony of Peter Sitclack (also spelled Sisscak), Transcript of the Anthracite Coal Strike Commission, December 17, 1902, Scranton, PA, NARA II, Vol. 22, Box 3, pp. 3178–88.

***whose interests are so inseparably allied*:** Testimony of John Mitchell, Transcript of the Anthracite Coal Strike Commission, November 14, 1902, Scranton, PA, NARA II, Vol. 2, Box 1, p. 9.

***the reasonableness and conservativeness of our officers*:** Testimony of John Mitchell, Transcript of the Anthracite Coal Strike Commission, November 15, 1902, Scranton, PA, NARA II, Vol. 3, Box 1, p. 223.

Mitchell brought union leaders, national organizers, and local union delegates to Shamokin: See Cornell, *The Anthracite Coal Strike of 1902*, 78–81; Proceedings of the Tri-District Convention, MG 109, Series 1, Subseries B, Box 1: Tri-District Convention Proceedings, Indiana University of Pennsylvania, Archives and Special Collections, Indiana, PA.

We'll be reasonable and try all conservative measures: UMW Resolution #10: "Whereas, in our opinion a strike at the present time (when the anthracite coal trade is in such a prosperous condition) would be detrimental to our organization and the country at large, therefore be it resolved, that we try all conservative measures to gain the concessions asked for, and if failing in this, that we refer our grievance to the Civic Arbitration Board…" Proceedings of the Tri-District Convention, MG 109, Series 1, Subseries B, Box 1: Tri-District Convention Proceedings, Indiana University of Pennsylvania, Archives and Special Collections, Indiana, PA.

***we will not deal with that organization*:** Statement of George Baer, Transcript of the Anthracite Coal Strike Commission, October 27, 1902, Scranton, PA, NARA II, Vol. 1, Box 1, p. 8.

***We'll save money on the wages*:** "All Anthracite Collieries Were Shut Down

Yesterday," *Miners' Journal*, May 13, 1902.

voted sixteen to twelve: "A Test Vote at Scranton was 16 to 12 in Favor of Strike," *Miners' Journal*, May 8, 1902.

oiling them up, and then burying them: "Miners Will Strike," *Miners' Journal*, May 10, 1902.

in four languages: Balch, *Our Slavic Fellow Citizens*, 292: "At one meeting, for instance, interpreters will address their people in Slovak, Polish, Bohemian and Lithuanian."

Miners, *after entering the mines at seven in the morning*: Testimony of W. H. Dettery, Transcript of the Anthracite Coal Strike Commission, December 3, 1902, Scranton, PA, NARA II, Vol. 10, Box 2, p. 1145.

***there is a standing one in Coxe Brothers Company*:** Testimony of W. H. Dettery, Transcript of the Anthracite Coal Strike Commission, December 3, 1902, p. 1150.

***you are blacklisted under that company for six months*:** Testimony of W. H. Dettery, Transcript of the Anthracite Coal Strike Commission, December 3, 1902, pp. 1151, 1171–72.

***A man has to take any kind of a place that is given him*:** Testimony of Paul Dunleavy, Transcript of the Anthracite Coal Strike Commission, December 8, 1902, p. 1748.

***I was informed by the people that works*:** Testimony of Henry Shovlin, Transcript of the Anthracite Coal Strike Commission, December 8, 1902, Scranton, PA, NARA II, Vol. 14, Box 3, p. 1792.

You all know Kate Burns, right?: See the full testimony of Kate Burns, Transcript of the Anthracite Coal Strike Commission, December 9, 1902, Scranton, PA, NARA II, Vol. 15, Box 3, pp. 1,982–90, and Andrew Chippie, Transcript of the Anthracite Coal Strike Commission, December 6, 1902, Scranton, PA, NARA II, Vol. 13, Box 3, pp. 1619–30.

***I did not apply any other place*:** Testimony of Mike Midlick, Transcript of the Anthracite Coal Strike Commission, December 3, 1902, p. 1209.

***In my experience a good practical miner*:** Testimony of W. H. Dettery, Transcript of the Anthracite Coal Strike Commission, December 3, 1902, pp. 1172–73.

***And you won't have it all learned then either*:** Testimony of John T. Strannix, Transcript of the Anthracite Coal Strike Commission, December 4, 1902, Scranton, PA, NARA II, Vol. 11, Box 2, p. 1263.

***I wish I was. I was once*:** Testimony of William Hill, Transcript of the Anthracite Coal Strike Commission, December 9, 1902, Scranton, PA, NARA II,

Vol. 15, Box 3, p. 2011.

***about 70 percent* of everyone in the asylum *has chronic rheumatism*:** Testimony of Dr. Eugene J. Butler, Transcript of the Anthracite Coal Strike Commission, November 21, 1902, Scranton, PA, NARA II, Vol. 8, Box 2, pp. 984–86.

the Jeddo miners vote unanimously: "Freeland's Delegates," *Freeland Tribune*, May 14, 1902, p. 1.

Chapter 2: A Miners' Timeline

***communication by water*:** John Fanning Watson, Annals of Philadelphia and Pennsylvania, in the Olden Time: Being a Collection of Memoirs, Anecdotes, and Incidents of the City and Its Inhabitants, and of the Earliest Settlements of the Inland Part of Pennsylvania, from the Days of the Founders, Embellished with Engravings, vol. 2 (Philadelphia: Pennington, 1844).

The phrase Walking Purchase: See Jeffrey Ostler, *Surviving Genocide: Native Nations and the United States from the American Revolution to Bleeding Kansas* (New Haven: Yale University Press, 2019).

say the courts: The court acknowledged that "the Delaware Nation once possessed aboriginal title to the land" (p. 21), which established it as a property claim extinguishable only by war or treaty, but in this case the court looked into the past and found a previously unknown mechanism for the legal dispossession of Native nations: the "sweeping authority allowing Thomas Penn to extinguish the Lenni Lenape tribes' aboriginal title." See Memorandum and Order, Nation v. Commonwealth of Pennsylvania, Civil Action No. 04-CV-166 (E.D. Pa. November 30, 2004).

***Conquest gives a title which the Courts of the conqueror cannot deny*:** Johnson & Graham's Lessee v. McIntosh, 21 U.S. 543 (1823).

the worst military defeat: In terms of lives lost, the defeat was three times greater than Wounded Knee. See Colin G. Calloway, *The Victory with No Name: The Native American Defeat of the First American Army* (Oxford: Oxford University Press, 2014).

the Era of Inland Commerce: See Christopher F. Jones, *Routes of Power: Energy and Modern America* (Cambridge: Harvard University Press, 2014); Earl E. Brown, *Commerce on Early American Waterways: The Transport of Goods by Arks, Rafts and Log Drives* (London: McFarland, 2010); Archer B. Hulbert, *The Paths of Inland Commerce: A Chronicle of Trial, Road, and Waterway* (New Haven: Yale University Press, 1920); Richmond E. Myers, "The Story of Transportation on the Susquehanna River," *New York History* 29, no. 2 (1948): 157–69; "History—Canals," Reading Company

Collection, 1520, Box 972, Hagley Library & Archive, Greenville, DE.

via the Morris Canal: On canal and waterway transport, see Robert J. Cornell, *The Anthracite Coal Strike of 1902* (New York: Russell & Russell, 1957), 5.

Laborers get eighty cents: G. O. Virtue, "The Anthracite Mine Laborers," *Bulletin of the Department of Labor* 13 (November 1897): 730.

The miners were blamed for their deaths: "Fatal Accident in a Coal Mine," Carbondale *Democrat*, June 14, 1845.

and nearly killed them all: "Explosion in a Coal Mine," *Perry County Democrat*, August 28, 1845, p. 2.

The miner was blamed for his death: "Fatal Accident," *Wilkes-Barre Advocate*, April 21, 1847, p. 2.

absconded with the miners' dues and was never seen again: On the Bates Union, see Kevin Kenny, *Making Sense of the Molly Maguires* (Oxford: Oxford University Press, 1998), 66–71; Grace Palladino, *Another Civil War: Labor, Capital, and the State in the Anthracite Regions of Pennsylvania, 1840–68* (Champaign: University of Illinois Press, 1990), 53; Cornell, *The Anthracite Coal Strike of 1902*, 13.

***and retain it for purposes of national defence*:** Robley D. Evans, "Reserve our Anthracite for our Navy," *The North American Review* 184, (1907): 246.

to more than a million tons by 1837: See Chandler Alfred, "Anthracite Coal and the Beginnings of the Industrial Revolution in the United States," *Business History Review* 46, no. 2 (Summer 1972): 158; Cornell, *The Anthracite Coal Strike of 1902*, 7.

absorbed the smaller, regional societies that preceded it: On the WBA and predecessor unions, see Virtue, "Anthracite Mine Laborers," 732; Andrew Roy, *A History of the Coal Miners of the United States: From the Development of the Mines to the Close of the Anthracite Strike of 1902, Including a Brief Sketch of Early British Miners* (New York: Press of JL Trauger Printing Company, 1907).

organize mine workers into a labor cartel: Harold W. Aurand, *Coalcracker Culture: Work and Values in Pennsylvania Anthracite, 1835–1935* (Selinsgrove: Susquehanna University Press, 2003), 83–84; Clifton K. Yearly Jr., *Enterprise and Anthracite: Economics and Democracy in Schuylkill County, 1820–1875* (Baltimore: Johns Hopkins University Press, 1961), 181–88.

and the strike collapsed: Harold W. Aurand, "The Workingmen's Benevolent Association," *Labor History* 7, no. 1 (1966): 19–34; Edward Pinkowski, *John Siney, The Miners' Martyr* (Philadelphia: Sunshine Press, 1963).

Provost Marshal Charlemagne Towers: Palladino, *Another Civil War*, 4.

***Their powers are general*:** Pennsylvania P. L. 225, 1865P provides for such policemen for railroad companies, the provisions of which were extended to owners, lessees or other persons in possession of collieries, furnaces and rolling mills by act of 1866, P.L. 99.

Progressive-Era reformers called for the abolition of the Coal and Iron Police: Letter from Musmanno to Governor Gifford Pinchot, January 28, 1931, Musmanno Collection, Coal and Iron Police Sub-group, Series II: Coal and Iron Police Controversy, Box 2, Folder 9, Duquesne University Archives, Pittsburgh, PA.

***their violence made men communists*:** Musmanno's Funeral Oration, Musmanno Collection, Coal and Iron Police Sub-group, Series II: Coal and Iron Police Controversy, Box 2, Folder 7: Duquesne University Archives, Pittsburgh, PA.

established a standard wage-basis pegged to the price of coal: See Harold Aurand, *From the Molly Maguires to the United Mine Workers: The Social Ecology of an Industrial Union, 1869–1897* (Philadelphia: Temple University Press, 1971).

Gowen stage-managed an industry-wide tripling of freight rates: Kevin Kenny, *Making Sense of the Molly Maguires* (Oxford: Oxford University Press, 1998), 136–52.

***Gowen, anticipating all this, secretly created a front company*:** Eliot Jones, *The Anthracite Coal Combination in the United States* (Cambridge: Harvard University Press, 1914), 30; Jules Bogen, *The Anthracite Railroads: A Study in American Railroad Enterprise* (New York: Ronald Press, 1927), 57.

a growing army of Pinkertons: see Kenny, *Making Sense of the Molly Maguires*, 109.

***The Ballad of the Blacklegs*:** Sung by the blacksmith Patrick Johnson of the Eagle Hill Colliery, in George Korson, *Minstrels of the Mine Patch: Songs and Stories of the Anthracite Industry* (State College: Penn State University Press, 2016), 222–24.

***of rendering voluntary aid to each other in case of trouble*:** Letter from Simon Wolverton to L. C. Smith, May 1, 1902, Coxe Family Mining Papers, 3005, Box 555, Folder 15, Historical Society of Pennsylvania, Philadelphia, PA.

***We Never Sleep*:** See James Mackay, *Allan Pinkerton: The First Private Eye* (New York: John Wiley & Sons, 1996).

***slightly less galling and crushing tool of enslavement*:** Frederick Douglass, Narrative; Address of Hon. Fred. Douglass, delivered before the National Convention of Colored Men, at Louisville, KY, September 24, 1883.

black dragons: Allan Pinkerton, *The Molly Maguires and the Detectives* (New York: G. W. Carleton & Co., 1877), 444.

They settled their sights on the Ancient Order of the Hibernians: Letter from McParland to Allan Pinkerton, October 10, 1873, Reading Company Collection, Box 979, Folder: Molly Maguires, 1864–1875, Hagley Library & Archive.

the vindicated majesty of law: The exact phrase appeared in newspapers throughout the region. See Kenny, *Making Sense of the Molly Maguires*, 263.

proof of my words: Peter Linebaugh, "The Day of the Rope," *Counterpunch*, June 21, 2007.

glowed at night from the light of buried blue flames: Testimony of W. W. Ruley, Transcript of the Anthracite Coal Strike Commission, February 2, 1903, Philadelphia, PA, NARA II, Vol. 48, Box 8, p. 8,240; Jay Parini, "Anthracite Country," in *Anthracite Country Poems* (New York: Random House, 1982).

explode spontaneously: Aurand, *Coalcracker Culture*, 24.

Rain carried culm into creeks: Peter Roberts, *Anthracite Coal Communities: A Study of the Demography, the Social, Educational and Moral Life of the Anthracite Region* (New York: Macmillan, 1904), 9.

operators sold small amounts of cut-rate bony coal: Victor R. Greene, *The Slavic Community on Strike: Immigrant Labor in Pennsylvania Anthracite* (Notre Dame: University of Notre Dame Press, 1968), 226, note 24.

with shovels and wheelbarrows: Aurand, *Coalcracker Culture*, 115.

peddled it on the streets: Frank Norris, "Life in the Mining Region: A Study in Strike Time of the Conditions of Living in Representative Mining Towns," in *Everybody's Magazine* 7 (July–December, 1902): 246; Greene, *The Slavic Community on Strike*, 185.

made the burning of smaller grades of anthracite feasible: Aurand, *Coalcracker Culture*, 44.

in shirtsleeves, even in winter, digging: Testimony of R. S. Mercur, Transcript of the Anthracite Coal Strike Commission, January 22, 1903, Philadelphia, PA, NARA II, Vol. 40, Box 6, p. 6660.

surpassed the revenue of minecoal: Testimony of Frank Hatcher, Transcript of the Anthracite Coal Strike Commission, January 30, 1903, Philadelphia, PA, NARA II, Vol. 47, Box 8, p. 8127.

into a mass of black flowing stuff: Roberts, *Anthracite Coal Communities*, 7.

to merge with the Coal Miners' and Laborers' National Progressive Union:

Virtue, "*Anthracite Mine Laborers*," 747; Aurand, *Coalcracker Culture*, 135–37.

entirely too much attention to Hungarian weddings: "Coal and Iron Police," *Wilkes-Barre Times Leader*, August 13, 1897.

We need better protection: "Coal and Iron Police," Wilkes-Barre *Times Leader*, August 13, 1897.

had them shipped to the Pardee company store: "The guns for the posse came from the [North Lehigh] coal and Iron Police Association, which is always prepared for an emergency. 'They were purchased through Mr. Smith and shipped to Mr. Markle for me, Mr. Bullock and Mr. Drake gave their consent." Testimony of Ario Pardee Platt, quoted in "Sheriff Martin and Deputies on Trial," Wilkes-Barre *Sunday Leader*, March 6, 1898, pp. 10–11. Martin testified that he didn't know who procured the Lattimer posse's guns or where they'd come from. See "The Trial of Martin and His Deputies," Wilkes-Barre *Weekly Times*, March 5, 1898. Deputy Harris, of the Lattimer Posse, testified that the guns for the Lattimer posse came from the Pardee company store. He identified eight members of the posse from among Pardee & Co. clerks and foremen. "The Trial of Martin and His Deputies," Wilkes-Barre *Weekly Times*, March 5, 1898, p. 6.

Ario Pardee Platt, the manager of the company store: "Mr. Platt admitted that he was secretary and treasurer of the Coal and Iron Police Association of which Mr. Pardee, Mr. Markle and all the coal companies were members. He said the guns came from New York. There were 50 breech loading rifles and 50 breech loading shot guns." Platt went on to explain that he offered them to Martin and was sworn into the posse on coal company property. Testimony of Ario Pardee Platt, quoted in "The Trial of Martin and His Deputies," Wilkes-Barre *Weekly Times*, March 5, 1898, p. 8; The Coxe Bros. & Co. clerk E. A. Oberrender, whom Sheriff Martin appointed as a "special deputy," wrote Martin on September 16 to "call for protection," which led Martin to expand the size of the posse, deputizing police from the North Lehigh Association. See Oberrender to Martin, September 16, 1897, Coxe Family Mining Papers, MG 3005, Box B, Unbound Letterbooks 1892–1905, HSP; "Guns of Lattimer," Wilkes-Barre *Sunday Leader*, March 6, 1898.

Sheriff James Martin deputized the entire North Lehigh Coal and Iron Police Association: Wilkes-Barre *Times Leader*, February 26, 1898, p. 6.

We won't leave it until we reach Lattimer: *Hazleton Sentinel*, September 13, 1897.

as I was afraid to run: *Hazleton Sentinel*, September 23, 1897.

We had no particular leader: *Hazleton Sentinel*, September 23, 1897.

Martin Rosko turned to run: *Hazleton Sentinel*, September 10, 1897.

Deputy William Raught shoot a man: *Hazleton Sentinel*, September 13, 1897; Wilkes-Barre *Sunday Leader*, September 26, 1897.

A deputy kicked Mike Cheslak: *Hazleton Sentinel*, September 23, 1897.

The coroner found that most had been shot in the back: *Hazleton Sentinel*, September 13, 1897.

Andrew Shabolick survived: *Hazleton Sentinel*, September 10, 1897.

John Kulich took a bullet to the stomach: *Hazleton Sentinel*, September 10, 1897.

T. Milner Morris, collected the rifles: Letter from Oberrender to Smith, September 14, 1897, Coxe Family Mining Papers, MG 3005, Folder 263, Box B, Historical Society of Pennsylvania.

***it seems to me that the larger and more powerful a labor organization is*:** Testimony of John Mitchell, Transcript of the Anthracite Coal Strike Commission, November 18, 1902, Vol. 5, Box 1, p. 528.

occupied the coalfields with an army of teetotalers: See Asa Earl Martin, "The Temperance Movement in Pennsylvania Prior to the Civil War," *The Pennsylvania Magazine of History and Biography* 49, no. 3 (1925): 195–230.

***Industrial harmony*, the temperance advocates explained:** Palladino, *Another Civil War*, 55.

***would speed up production probably at least ten percent*:** As quoted in Eli Cook, The Pricing of Progress: Economic Indicators and the Capitalization of American Life (Cambridge: Harvard University Press, 2017), 3.

one-quarter of the work force: Palladino, *Another Civil War*, 75.

unassimilable immigrant populations: "Arrests for drunkenness involved immigrant workers almost exclusively." Sidney L. Harring, *Policing a Class Society: The Experience of American Cities, 1865–1915* (Rutgers: Rutgers University Press, 1983), 173. See also M. Craig Brown and Barbara D. Warner, "Immigrants, Urban Politics, and Policing in 1900," *American Sociological Review* 57, no. 3 (June 1992): 294.

***a large number of the mine workers*:** Statement of H. C. Reynolds, Transcript of the Anthracite Coal Strike Commission, January 22, 1903, NARA II, Vol. 40, Box 6, pp. 6837–38.

***the hillsides of Pennsylvania*:** "Senator Wheeler," *Pittsburgh Sun-Telegraph*, February 7, 1928.

***no anarchists in the trades union movement*:** Testimony of John Mitchell, Transcript of the Anthracite Coal Strike Commission, November 18, 1902, p. 487.

immense meetings in every mining town: Cornell, *The Anthracite Coal Strike of 1902*, 140.

It is my opinion, Mitchell testified: Testimony of John Mitchell, Transcript of the Anthracite Coal Strike Commission, November 14, 1902, Scranton, PA, NARA II, Vol. 2, Box 1, p. 114.

when the powers that govern: Statement by John Mitchell, Thursday, May 15, 1902, Grand Opera House, Hazleton, PA, Series 2, Box 109: Minutes of the Joint Convention of Districts No. 1, 7, and 9, United Mine Workers of America, p. 83. John Mitchell Papers, Catholic University of America, Washington, DC.

They are *not receiving proper wages*: Statement by John Mitchell, May 15, 1902, Minutes of the Joint Convention, p. 84. John Mitchell Papers, Catholic University of America, Washington, DC.

Under no circumstances: "Will Not Recognize Mine-Workers' Union," Philadelphia *Times*, September 6, 1900.

called a region-wide strike in September 1900: Testimony of John Mitchell, Transcript of the Anthracite Coal Strike Commission, November 17, 1902, Scranton, PA, NARA II, Vol. 4, Box 1, pp. 353–35.

if an old man falls behind a strong man: Testimony of George Maxey, Transcript of the Anthracite Coal Strike Commission, January 14, 1903, Philadelphia, PA, NARA II, Vol. 33, Box 5, p. 5445.

Johnnie Mitchell's my boss: Testimony of W. G. Thomas, Superintendent for Black Diamond Coal Co., Transcript of the Anthracite Coal Strike Commission, January 23, 1903, Philadelphia, PA, NARA II, Vol. 41, Box 6, p. 7037.

delegates established four principal demands: Cornell, *The Anthracite Coal Strike of 1902*, 42, 248; Proceedings of the Joint Convention held at the Shamokin Opera House, March 18–24, 1902, Series 1, Subseries B, Box 1, Folder: Joint Convention (Districts 1, 7, 9), 1902, MG 109, Indiana University of Pennsylvania, Archives and Special Collections.

renders the operations of our mines possible: "Will the Hazleton Delegate Convention Order a Strike?" *Miners' Journal*, May 14, 1902.

destroy the corporation: Edward Sherwood Meade, "The Investor's Interest in the Demands of the Anthracite Miners," *The Annals of the American Academy of Political and Social Science* 21 (January 1903): 36.

the doctored books of the coal companies: Statement by John Mitchell, Thursday, May 15, 1902, Grand Opera House, Hazleton, PA.

crushed to death, drowned, or asphyxiated: Roberts, *Anthracite Coal*

Communities, 265.

***I am of the opinion*, he wrote to Mother Jones:** Quoted in Craig Phelan, *Divided Loyalties: The Public and Private Life of Labor Leader John Mitchell* (New York: SUNY Press, 1994), 160.

Chapter 3: On Strike Day in Hazelton

***They say they will go to Europe*:** "Will the Miners' Delegate Convention Order a Strike?" *Miners' Journal*, May 12, 1902.

climbed up to a second-story balcony: "Miners Will Vote on a Strike Today," *New York Times*, May 14, 1902, p. 1; "Waiting for a Decision," *Freeland Tribune*, May 14, 1902.

pasteboard boxes under their arms full of passenger pigeons: *Miners' Journal*, May 15, 1902.

***curling columns of black smoke*:** "Operators are Firm Despite Recent Threat of the Union," *Miners' Journal*, May 23, 1902.

***it was not arbitration the operators wanted*:** "Subordinate Officer," *New-York Tribune*, May 16, 1902, p. 4.

***As a matter of fact*, he proclaimed, *they won't live any other way*:** "Urged to Act Wisely," *New-York Tribune*, May 15, 1902, p. 4.

the crushing weight of taxes: see Emily Greene Balch, *Our Slavic Fellow Citizens* (New York: Charities Publication Committee, 1910), 51.

pushed from the eastern provinces: "The Hohenzollerns had been freeing the serfs in Germany, and incoming Germans bought estates in Poland and dispossessed their eastern neighbors. In addition the *szlachta*, the Polish landed gentry, lost much in the abortive midcentury revolution, and, heavily in debt, they sold more than a million acres to the Germans in the next forty years. The Prussian government financially encouraged the land transfer, and a movement of peoples began. The German landlords increasingly attracted the poorer Polish farmworkers from Russia and Galicia, while the Prussian Poles moved on to the more industrialized areas of western Europe and the United States." See Victor R. Greene, *The Slavic Community on Strike: Immigrant Labor in Pennsylvania Anthracite* (Notre Dame: University of Notre Dame Press, 1968), 19. See also Sylvia Jaworska, "Anti-Slavic Imagery in German Radical Nationalist Discourse at the Turn of the Twentieth Century: A Prelude to Nazi Ideology?" *Patterns of Prejudice* 45, no. 5 (2011): 435–52.

the debt of dead cattle and failed harvests: On the role of "bad harvests and cattle diseases causing debt," see Balch, *Our Fellow Slavic Citizens*, 101.

stew meat, baking beans, and root vegetables: For a description of life in the boardinghouses, see Peter Roberts, *Anthracite Coal Communities: A Study of the Demography, the Social, Educational and Moral Life of the Anthracite Region* (New York: Macmillan, 1904), 105; Testimony of Sophia Bolland, Transcript of the Anthracite Coal Strike Commission, December 3, 1902, Scranton, PA, NARA II, Volume 10, Box 2, p. 1,223.

a what's-on-hand existence: See Greene, *The Slavic Community on Strike*, 4–6.

dug potatoes from farmers' lands: Harold W. Aurand, *Coalcracker Culture: Work and Values in Pennsylvania Anthracite, 1835–1935* (Selinsgrove: Susquehanna University Press, 2003), 110.

Most never bought a winter coat: See Balch, *Our Fellow Slavic Citizens*, 375.

burned their waste in huge firepits: Greene, *The Slavic Community on Strike*, 43.

***They live underneath America*:** Balch, *Our Slavic Fellow Citizens*, 419.

***You are going to decide the most important movement*:** John Mitchell, First Session, Wednesday morning, May 14, 1902, John Mitchell Papers, Catholic University of America, Series 2, Box 109, Minutes of the Joint Convention of Districts No. 1, 7, and 9, United Mine Workers of America, Held in the Grand Opera House, Hazleton, Pennsylvania, May 14, 15, 16, 1902, p. 1.

the coal operators planned to infiltrate the convention: "It Looks Threatening," *New-York Tribune*, May 15, 1902, p. 1.

***At Shamokin*:** Delegate Edwards, Second Session, Wednesday afternoon, May 14, 1902, John Mitchell Papers, Catholic University of America, Series 2, Box 109, Minutes of the Joint Convention of Districts No. 1, 7, and 9, United Mine Workers of America, Held in the Grand Opera House, Hazleton, Pennsylvania, May 14, 15, 16, 1902, p. 14.

***Half of us have forgotten it*:** Unnamed Delegate, Second Session, Wednesday afternoon, May 14, 1902, p. 12.

A pickpocket worked his way through the crowd: "Delegates Vote For Strike," *New-York Tribune*, May 16, 1902.

***Didn't they just establish*:** Delegate Carne, Wednesday, Second Session, Wednesday afternoon, May 14, 1902, p. 14.

***Gentlemen, the password each delegate*:** Mitchell, Wednesday, Second Session, Wednesday afternoon, May 14, 1902, p. 16.

***up to the chair to be patient*:** Delegate Llewellyn, Wednesday, Second Session, Wednesday afternoon, May 14, 1902, p. 16.

the dance planned for that night: "On the Southside," Hazleton *Plain*

Speaker, May 15, 1902, p. 3.

partly on the unfair list: Delegate Bernard Duffy, Wednesday, Second Session, Wednesday afternoon, May 14, 1902, p. 16.

loafing on his front porch: "How News of the Strike is Handled," Hazleton *Plain Speaker*, May 19, 1902, p. 4.

Will they strike too?: "How News of the Strike is Handled," 4.

but he found no takers: "Betting on the Result," Hazleton *Plain Speaker*, May 15, 1902.

walk ten paces without someone stopping him: "Situation is Still Enveloped in Doubt," Hazleton *Plain Speaker*, May 15, 1902, p. 1.

They pledge to us their fraternal feelings: Mitchell, Third Session, Thursday morning, May 15, 1902, 9 a.m., p. 19.

Gentlemen, I presume the time has come: Mitchell, Third Session, Thursday morning, May 15, 1902, 9 a.m., p. 20.

good offices to bring about a peaceful solution: Mitchell, Third Session, Thursday morning, May 15, 1902, 9 a.m., p. 21.

refused *to concede anything*: Mitchell, Third Session, Thursday morning, May 15, 1902, 9 a.m., p. 22.

the committee was not unanimous: Mitchell, Third Session, Thursdaymorning, May 15, 1902, 9 a.m., p. 23.

Don't make this about the man who makes the argument: Mitchell, Third Session, Thursday morning, May 15, 1902, 9 a.m., p. 24.

I came here instructed to vote for a strike: Delegate Gallagher, Third Session, Thursday morning, May 15, 1902, 9 a.m., p. 25.

We won't have a union *if we desert the men*: Delegate Gallagher, Third Session, Thursday morning, May 15, 1902, 9 a.m., p. 25–26.

the time for speech-making had passed: Delegate Clark, Third Session, Thursday morning, May 15, 1902, 9 a.m., p. 27.

I don't see that we can do anything else: Delegate Davis, Third Session, Thursday morning, May 15, 1902, 9 a.m., p. 28.

I'm voting as instructed: Delegate Picton, Third Session, Thursday morning, May 15, 1902, 9 a.m., p. 29.

Focus on the motion: President Mitchell, Third Session, Thursday morning, May 15, 1902, 9 a.m., p. 29.

unless *it can be shown that concessions have been made*: Delegate John Taylor, Third Session, Thursday morning, May 15, 1902, 9 a.m., p. 29.

the most conservative labor leaders *the world has ever seen*: Delegate Llewellyn, Third Session, Thursday morning, May 15, 1902, 9 a.m., p. 29.

***attended a great many conventions*:** Delegate Watkins, Third Session, Thursday morning, May 15, 1902, 9 a.m., p. 30.

***Who opposes this?*:** Delegate Neil M'Kechnie, Third Session, Thursday morning, May 15, 1902, 9 a.m., pp. 30–31.

***I think the first of September would be a better time*:** Delegate Echersly, Third Session, Thursday morning, May 15, 1902, 9 a.m., pp. 31–32.

***If we have a strike that will last for six months*:** Delegate Mullarkey, Third Session, Thursday morning, May 15, 1902, 9 a.m., p. 32.

***Our local would be satisfied with that*:** Delegate Gilchrist, Third Session, Thursday morning, May 15, 1902, 9 a.m., p. 32.

***I have been in three or four strikes*:** Delegate John Reap, Third Session, Thursday morning, May 15, 1902, 9 a.m., p. 33.

***I'm willing to fight and die under Mitchell*:** Delegate Harper, Third Session, Thursday morning, May 15, 1902, 9 a.m., p. 34.

***What is there left for us to do?*:** Delegate Lewis, Third Session, Thursday morning, May 15, 1902, 9 a.m., p. 35.

***If anyone can convince me*:** Delegate Thomas, Third Session, Thursday morning, May 15, 1902, 9 a.m., p. 36.

who *would be better off later*: Delegate J. M. Loeffler, Third Session, Thursday morning, May 15, 1902, 9 a.m., p. 36.

***The time for deliberation, consideration and investigation*:** Delegate Peter McHale, Third Session, Thursday morning, May 15, 1902, 9 a.m., pp. 37–38.

***the fight has already begun*:** Delegate Price, Third Session, Thursday morning, May 15, 1902, 9 a.m., pp. 38–39.

***The challenge has been forced on us*:** Delegate Dempsey, Third Session, Thursday morning, May 15, 1902, 9 a.m., p. 40.

they *will turn their guns on the Local officers*: Delegate Dempsey, Third Session, Thursday morning, May 15, 1902, 9 a.m., pp. 39–41.

***the millions of tons of coal*:** Delegate Carne, Third Session, Thursday morning, May 15, 1902, 9 a.m., pp. 42–43.

***I have seen the day in the anthracite coal region*:** Delegate Gallagher, Third Session, Thursday morning, May 15, 1902, 9 a.m., pp. 45–46.

***That motion will not be entertained at this time*:** Mitchell, Third Session, Thursday morning, May 15, 1902, 9 a.m., p. 47.

the operators *will come out in the public press*: Delegate Hartlein, Third Session, Thursday morning, May 15, 1902, 9 a.m., pp. 47–50.

Hartlein had the right to say whatever he wanted to say: Mitchell, Third Session, Thursday morning, May 15, 1902, 9 a.m., p. 51.

***I do not believe it is good policy to strike now*:** Delegate Dempsey, Third Session, Thursday morning, May 15, 1902, 9 a.m., pp. 52–55.

***There was not a single union man in my place*:** Delegate Clauser, Third Session, Thursday morning, May 15, 1902, 9 a.m., p. 55.

***From morning till night one line after another*:** Delegate De Silva, Third Session, Thursday morning, May 15, 1902, 9 a.m., pp. 56–60.

***are just as staunch today*:** Delegate Evans, Third Session, Thursday morning, May 15, 1902, 9 a.m., p. 62.

***so much talk in the papers about Nichols being bull-headed*:** Delegate Nichols, Third Session, Thursday morning, May 15, 1902, 9 a.m., pp. 66–70.

***we have hungry wolves at our door*:** Delegate Loftus, Third Session, Thursday morning, May 15, 1902, 9 a.m., pp. 72–73.

someone will have to organize our children: Aurand, *Coalcracker Culture*, 97.

***To hear them one would think*:** Delegate Matti, Third Session, Thursday morning, May 15, 1902, 9 a.m., p. 76.

***Then they were suspended until further notice*:** Delegate Spaide, Third Session, Thursday morning, May 15, 1902, 9 a.m., p. 78.

in letters he would write: See Mary Harris Jones, *The Autobiography of Mother Jones* (Chicago: Charles H. Kerr Publishing Co., 1925); Cornell, *The Anthracite Coal Strike of 1902*, 91–92.

It has been a privilege, *a treasure*: Statement of John Mitchell, Fourth Session, Thursday afternoon, May 15, 1902, 9 a.m., p. 82.

***When once the miners met a crushing defeat*:** Statement of John Mitchell, Fourth Session, Thursday afternoon, May 15, 1902, 9 a.m., pp. 81–92.

Delegate Thomas motioned to make the vote unanimous: Motion of Delegate Thomas, Fourth Session, Thursday afternoon, May 15, 1902, 9 a.m., p. 103.

***I was instructed to ask if the miners*:** Wilberton Delegate, Fourth Session, Thursday afternoon, May 15, 1902, p. 119.

***are heart and soul with us*:** Delegate Carne, Fourth Session, Thursday afternoon, May 15, 1902, p. 120.

Why would we guard scabs: Delegate Davis, Fourth Session, Thursday afternoon, May 15, 1902, p. 120.

turn their guns on their fellow United Mine Workers: Unnamed Delegate, Fourth Session, Thursday afternoon, May 15, 1902, p. 121.

I don't think these men would have been killed: Delegate Miles Daugherty, Fourth Session, Thursday afternoon, May 15, 1902, p. 124.

police murder on command: Delegate John Fahy, Fourth Session, Thursday afternoon, May 15, 1902, p. 126.

If you think the operators are so much inclined: Delegate Jones, Fourth Session, Thursday afternoon, May 15, 1902, p. 126.

most just turned and raced to the telegraph wires: "Delegates Vote For Strike," *New-York Tribune*, May 16, 1902.

I have a wife and six children: "Pres. Mitchell Will Have his Headquarters at Wilkes-Barre," *Miners' Journal*, May 19, 1902.

Old men presented themselves at the poor houses: *Miners' Journal*, May 21, 1902.

Labor agents appeared at the train depots: Greene, *The Slavic Community on Strike*, 184.

they booked steamships back to Europe: *Philadelphia Inquirer*, May 20, 1902.

25,000 miners had returned to Europe: Cornell, *The Anthracite Coal Strike of 1902*, 95, note 2.

tent encampments near Blairsville: *Miners' Journal*, May 26, 1902.

a Schuylkill shipper was buying them all up: Greene, *The Slavic Community on Strike*, 185.

make off with their meat birds: Testimony of Brigadier General J. P. S. Gobin, Lt. Gov. of PA, Transcript of the Anthracite Coal Strike Commission, January 9, 1903, Philadelphia, PA, NARA II, Vol. 29, Box 5, p. 4633.

a great mischief of rats: "The Operators Will Have to Reduce the Working Hours," *Miners' Journal*, May 22, 1902.

The independent coal companies in Hazleton hatched a plan: Letter from L. C. Smith to E. A. Oberrender, May 12, 1902, Coxe Family Mining Papers, 3005, Box B: Letterbooks 1892–1905, Folder 260, HSP.

Chapter 4: They Called It the Flying Squadron

the state ran out of application forms: "Pres. Mitchell Will Have His Headquarters at Wilkes-Barre," *Miners' Journal*, May 19, 1902.

labor agents who walked up to men on the street: Testimony of James Gable, Coal & Iron Police, Transcript of the Anthracite Coal Strike Commission, February 2, 1903, Philadelphia, PA, NARA II, Vol. 48, Box 8, p. 8397.

The Philadelphia agencies advertised in the papers: Testimony of David Wilson, Transcript of the Anthracite Coal Strike Commission, February 2, 1903, Philadelphia, PA, NARA, II Vol. 48, Box 8, p. 8391.

with the same watchfulness maintained over camps**:** Opening Statement of H. C. Reynolds, Attorney Representing the Independent Operators, Transcript of the Anthracite Coal Strike Commission, January 22, 1903, Philadelphia, PA, NARA II, Vol. 40, Box 6, p. 6834.

They installed electric light plants: Testimony of J. G. Hayes, Superintendent of Peoples Coal Co., Transcript of the Anthracite Coal Strike Commission, January 23, 1903, Philadelphia, PA, NARA II, Vol. 41, Box 6, p. 7043.

they built barracks and commissaries: Testimony of George O. Thomas, Inside Foreman for Clear Spring Coal Co., Transcript of the Anthracite Coal Strike Commission, January 23, 1903, Philadelphia, PA, NARA II, Vol. 41, Box 6, p. 6,934; Testimony of Ario Pardee Platt, Purchasing Agent for A. Pardee and Flying Squadron Trooper, Transcript of the Anthracite Coal Strike Commission, January 27, 1903, Philadelphia, PA, NARA II, Vol. 44, Box 7, p. 7,493.

the Philadelphia and Reading Coal and Iron Company had an army of 350 private police: "Policemen," William A. Stone Papers, 1898–1903, MG-181, Box 2: Executive Correspondence, Folder: Executive Correspondence, 1902; Coal & Iron Police, Lists of Policemen and Companies re: Anthracite Coal Strike.

with nearly five thousand private cops in the coalfields: "Policemen appointed by Governor," Samuel W. Pennypacker Papers MG-171, Box 20: Executive Correspondence, commissions, Folder 2: Executive Correspondence, 1904–05, Commissions Coal & Iron Police Pennsylvania State Archives, Harrisburg, PA.

relations with the miners *were very pleasant*: Testimony of W. A. May, Transcript of the Anthracite Coal Strike Commission, January 13, 1903, Philadelphia, PA, NARA II, Vol. 32, Box 5, p. 5,258; Statement of J. R. Wilson, Attorney for the Delaware, Lackawanna & Western Railroad Co., Transcript of the Anthracite Coal Strike Commission, January 17, 1903, Philadelphia, PA, NARA II, Vol. 36, Box 6, p. 6001; Statement of James Torrey, Attorney for Delaware & Hudson Co., Transcript of the Anthracite Coal Strike Commission, January 10, 1903, Philadelphia, PA, NARA II, Vol. 30, Box 5 p. 4716.

dissatisfaction amongst the men**:** Statement of Everett Warren, Lawyer for

Hillside Coal & Iron Co., Transcript of the Anthracite Coal Strike Commission, January 13, 1903, Philadelphia, PA, NARA II, Vol. 32, Box 5, p. 5227.

desire for work: Statement of William Taylor, Lawyer for St. Clair Coal Co., Transcript of the Anthracite Coal Strike Commission, January 29, 1903, Philadelphia, PA, NARA II, Vol. 46, Box 7, p. 7892.

a spirit of insubordination: Testimony of Victor L. Peterson, Superintendent of Hillside Coal Co., Transcript of the Anthracite Coal Strike Commission, January 15, 1903, Philadelphia, PA, NARA II, Vol. 34, Box 6, p. 5470.

doesn't appreciate or understand our institutions: Statement of H. C. Reynolds, Transcript of the Anthracite Coal Strike Commission, January 22, 1903, NARA II, Vol. 40, Box 6, p. 6837.

unmanly, un-American, and un-Christian union leaders: "The Manly Thing," *Scranton Tribune*, June 12, 1902.

free American life makes necessary: Statement of H. C. Reynolds, Transcript of the Anthracite Coal Strike Commission, January 22, 1903, p. 6838.

gross agitators: Letter from R. M. Olyphant, President of Delaware & Hudson, to Charles C. Rose, Superintendent, Delaware & Hudson, Testimony of Charles C. Rose, Transcript of the Anthracite Coal Strike Commission, January 10, 1903, Philadelphia, PA, NARA II, Vol. 30, Box 5, p. 4729.

secure control of the government: Statement of James Torrey, Transcript of the Anthracite Coal Strike Commission, January 10, 1903, Philadelphia, PA, NARA II, Vol. 30, Box 5, p. 4,711; Cornell, *The Anthracite Coal Strike of 1902*, 131.

They won't listen: Testimony of William Allen, Inside Division Superintendent with Elk Hill Coal Co., Transcript of the Anthracite Coal Strike Commission, January 16, 1903, Philadelphia, PA, NARA II, Vol. 35, Box 6, p. 5777.

Johnny Mitchell is my boss: Cornell, *The Anthracite Coal Strike of 1902*, 73.

Don't you know you're a scab?: Testimony of John F. Cummings, Division Outside Foreman for Scranton Coal Co., Transcript of the Anthracite Coal Strike Commission, January 17, 1903, Philadelphia, PA, NARA II, Vol. 36, Box 6, p. 5985.

sleigh rides on demand: Testimony of William Allen, Inside Division Superintendent with Elk Hill Coal Co., Transcript of the Anthracite Coal Strike Commission, January 16, 1903, pp. 5774–77.

use some very mean names against us: Testimony of John F. Cummings, Division Outside Foreman for Scranton Coal Co., Transcript of the Anthracite

Coal Strike Commission, January 17, 1903, p. 5997.

To hell with the union: Testimony of Gabriel Evans, Transcript of the Anthracite Coal Strike Commission, February 5, 1903, Philadelphia, PA, NARA II, Vol. 51, Box 9, p. 9142.

belligerency and fearlessness: Greene, *The Slavic Community on Strike*, 97.

until his kidney ruptured: Testimony of William Jenkins, Engineer with Lehigh & Wilkes-Barre Coal Co., Transcript of the Anthracite Coal Strike Commission, January 6, 1903, Philadelphia, PA, NARA II, Vol. 26, Box 4, p. 3977.

When scabs took their jobs, they chased after them: Testimony of John L. Williams, Civil & Mining Engineer for Lehigh & Wilkes-Barre Coal Co., Transcript of the Anthracite Coal Strike Commission, January 6, 1903, Philadelphia, PA, NARA II, Vol. 7, Box 2, pp. 3925–26; Testimony of Rev. Peter Roberts, Transcript of the Anthracite Coal Strike Commission, November 20, 1902, Scranton, PA, NARA II, Vol. 7, Box 2, p. 857; "Strikers on the Rampage," *New York Times*, August 10, 1887.

They stormed jails and staged jailbreaks: Greene, *The Slavic Community on Strike*, 172.

Others chased them out with clubs and axes: Letter from E. A. Oberrender to L. C. Smith, October 3, 1900, Coxe Family Mining Papers, 3005, Box 557, Folder 3, HSP.

recruitment of private police and scabs: See testimony of Charles H. Schadt, Lackawanna County Sheriff, Transcript of the Anthracite Coal Strike Commission, January 6, 1903, Philadelphia, PA, NARA II, Vol. 26, Box 4 p. 3949; *Miners' Journal*, May 19 1902, "Pres. Mitchell Will Have his Headquarters at Wilkes-Barre"; "Situation Unchanged in the Anthracite Coalfields," *Miners' Journal*, May 31, 1902.

sheriff offered five times the miners' wages: "Operators Preparing for a Long Conflict," *Miners' Journal*, June 11, 1902.

now saw all the effigies hanging: Cornell, *The Anthracite Coal Strike of 1902*, pp, 144–5.

scores of collieries were forced to shut down their pumps: "May Ask for State and Federal Protection," *Miners' Journal*, June 7, 1902.

***Avoid being drawn into quarrels*:** Testimony of George W. Hartlein, UMW District 9 Secretary, Transcript of the Anthracite Coal Strike Commission, February 5, 1903, NARA II, Vol. 51, Box 9, pp. 9, 111–12.

***Scabs must leave town, Death to Scabs*:** One banner read: "The scabs of Miners Mills and Plains. Daniel Powell, Willie Powell, Johnie Jones, J. J. Jones,

Johnie Lewis, Fleck Walker, John George Ayers, John Henry Thomas, Tommie Jenkins, a greenhorn blackleg, James Gray, a Blackleg Sneak, Jack Thomson, Tomie Roberts, Willie Roberts, John Foot Sorber, Steve Sandison, Owen Williams, Dobble, a blackleg scab, Albert Harws, a blackleg, Simons the scab, Charlie Olphant Cook a scab . . . Signed: Wint. Oplinger, Jim Barret, Joe Athey, Jim O'Brien": Testimony of Daniel Powell, Miners' Mills Driver boss, Transcript of the Anthracite Coal Strike Commission, January 8, 1903, Philadelphia, PA, NARA II, Vol. 24, Box 4, p. 3769; See also "They Return," *Miners' Journal*, June 4, 1902; Testimony of Lillie Stephenson, Spouse of Assistant Breaker Foremen at Silver Creek Colliery, and Mrs. Robert Robinson, spouse of Brookside Colliery Engineer, Transcript of the Anthracite Coal Strike Commission, January 8, 1903, Philadelphia, PA, NARA II, Vol. 28, Box 4, pp. 4321, 4325.

stuffed with plantain leaves and garden rubbish: Testimony of William Gardner, Weighmaster for Penn. Coal Co., Transcript of the Anthracite Coal Strike Commission, December 19, 1902, Philadelphia, PA, NARA II, Vol. 24, Box 4 p. 3773.

They strung banners across bridges: Testimony of David Powell, Driver Boss, Transcript of the Anthracite Coal Strike Commission, December 19, 1902, Scranton, PA, NARA II, Vol. 24, Box 4, p. 3767.

Handel's "Dead March": "They Return," *Miners' Journal*, June 4, 1902.

Striking breaker boys on bikes ferried messages back and forth: Testimony of Albert C. Leisnering, Superintendent of the Upper Lehigh Coal Co., Transcript of the Anthracite Coal Strike Commission, January 27, 1902, Philadelphia, PA, NARA II, Vol. 44, Box 7, p. 7576.

***One of the women came at me with a club*:** Testimony of John Frederick, Bliss Colliery Engineer, Transcript of the Anthracite Coal Strike Commission, December 18, 1902, Scranton, PA, NARA II, Vol. 23, Box 3, p. 3566.

and marched him out of town: Testimony of Thomas Whildin, General Inside Foreman for Lehigh Coal & Navigation Co., Transcript of the Anthracite Coal Strike Commission, January 28, 1903, Philadelphia, PA, NARA II, Vol. 45, Box 7, p. 7705; Testimony of John Mitchell, President of the United Mine Workers, Transcript of the Anthracite Coal Strike Commission, November 17, 1902, Scranton, PA, NARA II, Vol. 4, Box 1, pp. 416–17.

he'd find a freshly dug grave in his yard: Cornell, *The Anthracite Coal Strike of 1902*, 145.

***SCAB HOUSE*:** "Daubed a House," Hazleton *Plain Speaker*, June 13, 1902.

Polish women threatened to: Roberts, *Anthracite Coal Communities*, 287; Palladino, *Another Civil War*, 99–100.

Strikers set the Hollenback and Stanton colliery stockades on fire: Testimony of Eugene Lawson, Company Store Keeper for Lehigh & Wilkes-Barre Coal Co., Transcript of the Anthracite Coal Strike Commission, January 7, 1903, Philadelphia, PA, NARA II, Vol. 27, Box 4, pp. 4, 195–97; Statement of A. H. McClintock, Attorney for Lehigh & Wilkes-Barre Coal Co., Transcript of the Anthracite Coal Strike Commission, January 22, 1903, Philadelphia, PA, NARA II, Vol. 40, Box 6, p. 6734.

a squad of marching women armed with long sticks: "Women Held up Supt. Kudlick," *Hazleton Plain Speaker*, June 9, 1902.

***I could not move a column of my troops*:** Testimony of John P. S. Gobin, Brigadier General of N. P. S. & Lt. Gov. of PA, Transcript of the Anthracite Coal Strike Commission, January 9, 1902, Philadelphia, PA, NARA II, Vol. 29, Box 5, pp. 4593–94.

***Each parade makes them stronger*:** "Mother Jones at Hazleton," *Miners' Journal*, August 13, 1902.

spiked train tracks, cocked train switches, and bridges on fire: Testimony of Davis L. Jenkins, Coal & Iron Police for the Pennsylvania and Reading Coal and Iron Co., Transcript of the Anthracite Coal Strike Commission, January 7, 1902, Philadelphia, PA, NARA II, Vol. 27, Box 4, Volume 27, pp. 4309–12.

began mysteriously blowing up: "They blew the porch down and caved the side of the house in, smashed all the windows, and lifted the wife and three children out of the bed." Testimony of Richard Partfit, Gilberton Fireboss, Transcript of the Anthracite Coal Strike Commission, January 7, 1902, Philadelphia, PA, NARA II, Vol. 27, Box 4, p. 4270.

triggering a seventy-ton avalanche that blocked the railroad tracks: Testimony of Lawrence Jenkins, Luzerne County Deputy Sheriff, Transcript of the Anthracite Coal Strike Commission, January 8, 1903, Philadelphia, PA, NARA II, Vol. 28, Box 4, p. 4514.

after an explosion destroyed the Lehigh and Wilkes-Barre's Jersey Annex dam: Testimony of D. C. Tiffany, Outside Foreman, Lehigh & Wilkes-Barre Coal Co., Transcript of the Anthracite Coal Strike Commission, January 7, 1903, Philadelphia, PA, NARA II, Vol. 27, Box 4, p. 4101.

woke up one night to the sound of explosions: Testimony of William J. Richards, General Superintendent of Lehigh & Wilkes-Barre Coal Co., Transcript of the Anthracite Coal Strike Commission, January 22, 1903, Philadelphia, PA, NARA II, Vol. 40, Box 6, p. 6772.

and drove the train into the back of another at full speed: Testimony of Thomas Franklin, Conductor for the Central Railroad of New Jersey, Transcript of the Anthracite Coal Strike Commission, January 6, 1903,

Philadelphia, PA, NARA II, Vol. 26, Box 4, p. 4048.

***Ye vile dogs of SATAN*:** Testimony of Erwin E. Finch, Special Officer for Lehigh & Wilkes-Barre Coal Co., Transcript of the Anthracite Coal Strike Commission, January 7, 1903, Philadelphia, PA, NARA II, Volume 27, Box 4, p. 4151.

The Brotherhood of Railroad Firemen announced: "Waiting for Answer From the President," *Miners' Journal*, June 6, 1902.

The barbers of North Scranton began refusing: "Cannot Assist," *Miners' Journal*, June 16, 1902.

***In past years we have had considerable secret service work*:** Letter from Simon Wolverton to L. C. Smith, May 1, 1902, Coxe Family Mining Papers, MG 3305, Folder 15, Box 555, HSP.

the Irish had *the run of the jail*: Letters from H. W. Bearce, Pinkerton Agent, to E. A. Oberrender, November 2 and 18, 1900, Coxe Family Mining Papers, 3005, Box 555, Folder 15, Historical Society of Pennsylvania, Philadelphia, PA.

***We want to hold the power of employing and arming men*:** Letter from Simon Wolverton to L. C. Smith, May 1, 1902.

***Throw aside all ordinary work*:** Letter from L. C. Smith to E. A. Oberrender, May 24, 1902, Coxe Family Mining Papers, 3005, Box 654, Folder 25, HSP.

***two trains of cars ready*:** Testimony of Ario Pardee Platt, Secretary and Treasurer for North Lehigh Association and purchasing Agent for Pardee & Co., Transcript of the Anthracite Coal Strike Commission, January 27, 1903, p. 7508.

***get together a force of reliable men*:** Testimony of Willard Young, Transcript of the Anthracite Coal Strike Commission, January 27, 1903, p. 7527.

he hired Ario Pardee Platt: Testimony of Ario Pardee Platt, Transcript of the Anthracite Coal Strike Commission, January 27, 1903, p. 7506.

***any point in the territory within twenty or twenty-five miles*:** Testimony of Ario Pardee Platt, Transcript of the Anthracite Coal Strike Commission, January 27, 1903, p. 7504.

nothing like the restructured North Lehigh Association existed anywhere: See Gary Jones, "American Cossacks: The Pennsylvania Department of State Police and Labor, 1890–1917" (PhD diss, Lehigh University, 1997); Sidney L. Harring, *Policing a Class Society: The Experience of American Cities, 1865–1915* (Rutgers: Rutgers University Press, 1983); Kristian Williams, *Our Enemies in Blue: Police and Power in America* (Oakland: AK Press, 2015); the Musmanno Collection, Coal and Iron Police, Series II:

Coal and Iron Police Controversy, Box 2, Folder 13, Duquesne University Archives, Pittsburgh, PA.

What Young didn't know was that the union had been posting sentries: Letter from Craig Loose to E. A. Oberrender, June 9, 1902, Coxe Family Mining Papers, 3005, Box 560, Folder 12, HSP.

***The men were all sitting there*:** Testimony of Daniel T. McKelvey, Transcript of the Anthracite Coal Strike Commission, February 3, 1903, Philadelphia, PA, NARA II, Vol. 49, Box 8, p. 8447.

***Are you not workingmen yourselves?*:** Testimony of RJ Beamish, Newspaper Reporter for *The North American*, Transcript of the Anthracite Coal Strike Commission, February 2, 1902, Philadelphia, PA, NARA II, Vol. 48, Box 8, p. 8337.

the strikers parading up and down the street: "Hotel Girls Join Strikers," *Miners' Journal*, June 3, 1902.

***You're not doing what you're supposed to do*:** Testimony of Willard Young, Transcript of the Anthracite Coal Strike Commission, January 27, 1903, p. 7527.

Incite a riot: Oberrender's notes, Coxe Family Mining Papers, 3005, Box 655, Folder 24, HSP; "Wanted Strikers to Riot," *Pottsville Republican*, June 9, 1902, p. 1; "Has Collapsed," Hazleton *Plain Speaker*, June 13, 1902.

***and I only had limited time*:** Testimony of Willard Young, Transcript of the Anthracite Coal Strike Commission, January 27, 1903, p. 7527.

Smith ordered Oberrender to have Duffy arrested: Letter from Oberrender to S. H. Karcher, June 3 1902, Coxe Family Mining Papers, 3005, Box 560, Folder 9, HSP.

***to get the poor miner to buckle*:** Testimony of Daniel T. McKelvey, Transcript of the Anthracite Coal Strike Commission, February 3, 1903, pp. 8441–3.

fire those he suspected of holding union sympathies: "Drifton Guards Dismissed," *Miners' Journal*, June 13, 1902; "Wanted Strikers to Riot," *Pottsville Republican*, June 9, 1902; Letter from Oberrender to Smith, June 21, 1902, Coxe Family Mining Papers, 3005, Box 555, Folder 13, HSP; *Pottsville Republican*, June 9, 1902, "Wanted Strikers to Riot"; Letter from Oberrender to Smith, September 30, 1902, Coxe Family Mining Papers, 3005, Letterpress Volume 246, HSP; Letter from Oberrender to Wolverton, June 15, 1901, Coxe Family Mining Papers, 3005, Box 555, Folder 10, HSP; Letter from Oberrender to Smith, May 31, 1902, Coxe Family Mining Papers, 3005, Box 560, Folder 4, HSP.

Chicago Haymarket affair: In May 1886, during a labor rally in Chicago's Haymarket Square, a bomb exploded in the crowd, killing seven cops.

Police arrested eight people, including August Spies, editor of the anarchist newspaper *Arbeiter Zeitung*, who had been speaking at the rally when the bomb went off. It had been Bartholomew Flynn who'd searched the *Arbeiter*'s office and who said, on the stand, that he'd "found a lot of fuses, some caps, some dynamite sticks in Mr. Spies' drawer." Sixteen months later, on November 11, 1887, Spies and three other men were hanged to death. See letter from L. C. Smith to E. A. Oberrender, June 5, 1902 and from Oberrender to McClintock, June 7, 1902, Coxe Family Mining Papers, 3005, Box 560, Folder 12, HSP; Testimony of Bartholomew Flynn, Illinois v. August Spies et al. trial transcript no. 1, 1886 July 22, Volume J, 118–26, Chicago Historical Society, Haymarket Affair Digital Collection; Letter from Craig and Loose, Attorneys at Law, to E. A. Oberrender, June 9, 1902, Coxe Family Mining Papers, 3005, Box 560, Folder 12, HSP.

the Secret Service Department: Letter from Smith to Oberrender, May 24, 1902, Coxe Family Mining Papers, MG 3005, Box 654, Folder 25, HSP; Letter from H. W. Bearce, Pinkerton Agent to E. A. Oberrender, November 18, 1900, Coxe Family Mining Papers, 3005, Box 556, Folder 23, HSP; Letter from E. A. Oberrender to R. J. Linden, Pinkerton Agent, July 25, 1884, Coxe Family Mining Papers, 3005, Box 564, Folder 9, HSP; Letter from E. A. Oberrender to Malcolm Franklin, Benjamin Franklin Detective Agency, March 4, 1902, Box 654, Folder 3, HSP; See Letter from J. H. Remington letter to Rohland, and Sweeny, July 25, 1901, Coxe Family Mining Papers, 3005, Box 558, Folder 21, HSP; Oberrender's Notes, August 6, 1902, Coxe Family Mining Papers, 3005, Box 560, Folder 23, HSP; Affidavit of John James, July 1, 1902, Coxe Family Mining Papers, 3005, Box 561, Folder 4, HSP. Letter from E. A. Oberrender to S. D. Warriner, Supt. Lehigh Valley Coal Company, January 21, 1902, Coxe Family Mining Papers, 3005, Box B: Unbound Letterbooks, 1892–1905, Folder 260, HSP.

Billy Evans of the *Hazleton Sentinel*: August 1902 itinerary, Coxe Family Mining Papers, 3005, July 1 1902, Box 560, Folder 3, HSP.

his willingness to perjure himself for a fee: Letter from John James to E. A. Oberrender, n.d., Box 560, Folder 23; Oberrender's Notes, August 6, 1902; Affidavit of John James, July 1, 1902, Box 561, Folder 4; Letter from L C. Smith to E. A. Oberrender, July 23, 1902, Box 520, Folder 23, Coxe Family Mining Papers, 3005, HSP.

and to keep track of their movements: Wassmer had been surveilling the strikers since the start of the strike, and the Flying Squadron relied on his daily updates to Smith. Affidavit of Isaac Eckert, July 1, 1902; Affidavit of Barth Flynn, July 1 1902; Affidavit of John Rohland, July 1, 1902, Coxe Family Mining Papers, 3005, Box 560, Folder 20, HSP.

***avenged*:** Letter from Smith to Oberrender, July 8, 1902, Coxe Family Mining

Papers, 3005, Box 561, Folder 4, HSP; Testimony of Willard Young, Transcript of the Anthracite Coal Strike Commission, January 27, 1903, p. 7,535; Affidavit of John Rohland, July 1, 1902, Coxe Family Mining Papers, 3005, Box 560, Folder 20, HSP.

they found the Flying Squadron waiting for them: Testimony of Willard Young, Transcript of the Anthracite Coal Strike Commission, January 27, 1903, pp. 7,536–37; Transcript of Commonwealth of Pennsylvania v. William Gelgot, John Waskevicz, John Shrader and John (alias Duff) Shovlin, Wilkes-Barre City Court, Wednesday, July 2, 1902, Coxe Family Mining Papers, 3005, Box 560, Folder 15, HSP.

read the riot act: Testimony of Isaac Eckert, p. 14, Commonwealth of Pennsylvania v. William Gelgot, John Waskevicz, John Shrader, and John (Duff) Shovlin, Coxe Family Mining Papers, 3005, Box 560, Folder 15, HSP.

***sons of bitches*:** Testimony of Charles Rohland, p. 4, Commonwealth of Pennsylvania v. William Gelgot, John Waskevicz, John Shrader, and John (Duff) Shovlin, Coxe Family Mining Papers, 3005, Box 560, Folder 15, HSP.

***They have no more right on the street*:** Testimony of Isaac Eckert, p. 15, Commonwealth of Pennsylvania v. William Gelgot, John Waskevicz, John Shrader, and John (Duff) Shovlin, Coxe Family Mining Papers, 3005, Box 560, Folder 15, HSP.

if he got him alone in Freeland: Testimony of Charles Rohland, p. 4, Commonwealth of Pennsylvania v. William Gelgot, John Waskevicz, John Shrader, and John (Duff) Shovlin, Coxe Family Mining Papers, 3005, Box 560, Folder 15, HSP.

***What right do you have*:** Testimony of Isaac Eckert, p. 16-17, Commonwealth of Pennsylvania v. William Gelgot, John Waskevicz, John Shrader, and John (Duff) Shovlin, Coxe Family Mining Papers, 3005, Box 560, Folder 15, HSP.

railroaded the four strikers to Weatherly: "Riots in the Coalfields" and "The Clash at Drifton," *Miners' Journal*, July 3, 1902; "Heavy Rains are Flooding the Anthracite Coal Mines," *Miners' Journal*, July 4, 1902.

in city after city: "Riots in the Coalfields."

and setting bonfires at night: "Heavy Rains are Flooding the Anthracite Coal Mines."

the strikers declared a boycott: Testimony of James Fahey, Special Agent of the Lackawanna Railroad Co., Transcript of the Anthracite Coal Strike Commission, December 19, 1902, Scranton, PA, NARA II, Vol. 24, Box 4, p. 3,646; Testimony of Christopher McDermott, Fire Boss for Penn. Coal Co., Transcript of the Anthracite Coal Strike Commission, December 19,

1902, Scranton, PA, NARA II, Vol. 24, Box 4, p. 3770.

boycotted scabs fired from teaching jobs: "Thomas Coogan, engineer at Racket Brook was compelled to stop by a threat that his sister would be discharged from her place as a school teacher." See Testimony of John Mitchell, Transcript of the Anthracite Coal Strike Commission, November 17, 1902, pp. 372–400; Oberrender's Notes, August 6, 1902.

from Catholic priests: "I was called to Lansford to bury a man belonging to our faith, the Protestant Lutheran, Slavic. I came up on the 16th of September and when I had got there nobody was there. . . . I was met by a committee who told me I should not bury that man. . . . I asked why. They said, 'He is a scab.'" Testimony of Carl Hauser, Lutheran priest from Freeland, Transcript of the Coal Strike Commission, January 9, 1903, Philadelphia, PA, NARA II, Vol. 29, Box 5, p. 4558.

***John Foote, the bloody scab; Albert Catley's Last Chance*:** Catley was also blacklisted by the grocer, milk man, and the laundry: Testimony of Albert Catley, Assistant Inside Foreman, Transcript of the Anthracite Coal Strike Commission, January 7, 1903, Philadelphia, PA, NARA II, Vol. 27, Box 4, p. 4,218; John Foote's cow was killed and his grocer was told he'd be tarred and feathered if he kept selling to Foote. Testimony of John Foote, Engineer for Delaware & Hudson Co., Transcript of the Anthracite Coal Strike Commission, January 7, 1903, Philadelphia, PA, NARA II, Vol. 28, Box 4, p. 4482.

***don't you think you should come out*:** Letter from E. A. Oberrender to L. C. Smith, June 30, 1902, Coxe Family Mining Papers, Box 560, Folder 11, HSP.

***I work at anything Rohland has charge of*:** Letter from E. A. Oberrender to L. C. Smith, June 30, 1902.

***anything else we can use legally*:** Letter from L. C. Smith to E. A. Oberrender, June 26, 1902, Coxe Family Mining Papers, 3005, Box 560, Folder 11, HSP.

***Then take it out of me*:** Letter from E. A. Oberrender to L. C. Smith, June 30, 1902.

***We are the right*:** Report of Albin Wassmer, June 6, 1902, Coxe Family Mining Papers, 3005, Box 561, Folder 4, HSP.

I *met a mob of about 300 people*: Affidavit of Albin Wassmer, July 1, 1902, Coxe Family Mining Papers, 3005, Box 561, Folder 4, HSP.

a railway fireman stopped by the crowd: Testimony of Willard Young, Chief of the Flying Squadron, Transcript of the Anthracite Coal Strike, p. 7526.

***A man named Mulraney caught Wassmer*:** Affidavit of Joe Reynolds, Coxe Family Mining Papers, 3005, July 1, 1902, Box 561, Folder 4, HSP.

preserved the peace and good order: "Evidence by Captain B. Flynn against Dan Mulreany," July 1, 1902, Coxe Family Mining Papers, 3005, Box 560, Folder 20, HSP.

thugs: Affidavit of Charles Rohland; Affidavit of A.F. Harger, Coxe Family Mining Papers, 3005, 1 July 1902, Box 560, Folder 20, HSP.

you have *to deserve it*: Oberrender's Notes, August 6, 1902, Coxe Family Mining Papers, 3005, Box 560, Folder 23, HSP.

Boyles saloon where Wassmer: Affidavit of John James, July 1, 1902, Box 561, Folder 4, HSP.

Oberrender hired James: Oberrender's Notes, August 6, 1902.

A sailor named Franch: Oberrender's notes, July 15, 1902, Coxe Family Mining Papers, 3005, Box 561, Folder 4, HSP.

push the matter faster: Letter from L. C. Smith to E. A. Oberrender, July 8, 1902, Coxe Family Mining Papers, 3005, Box 561, Folder 4, HSP.

I'm very much disappointed in your work: Oberrender's Notes, August 6, 1902.

the feeling of the people about Freeland: Oberrender's Notes, August 6, 1902.

a riot, a mob armed with clubs: Oberrender's Notes, July 1, 1902, Coxe Family Mining Papers, 3005, Letterpress Volume 246, HSP.

under bond for trial: Oberrender's Notes, July 1, 1902.

crying for bread: Testimony of John Harvilla, Boiler Operator for Coxe Bros. & Co., Transcript of the Anthracite Coal Strike Commission, January 9, 1903, pp. 4555–56.

We want to fight it if we can: "See Mr. Rohland and get the evidence which will determine whether we have a case or not. We want to fight it if we can." Handwritten note below letter from John Rohland to L. C. Smith, August 27, 1902.

and shortly after I reached home a Jew from Hazleton: Letter from E. A. Oberrender to L. C. Smith, August 27, 1902, Coxe Family Mining Papers, 3005, Box 561, Folder 13, HSP.

a lot of boys and some men with them came to my place: Oberrender Notes, September 2, 1902, Coxe Family Mining Papers, 3005, Box 561, Folder 22, HSP.

a shotgun blast struck me in the face: Oberrender Notes, September 1, 1902, Coxe Family Mining Papers, 3005, Box 561, Folder 22, HSP.

Leave me alone: Testimony of John Harvilla, Boiler Operator for Coxe Bros.

& Co., Transcript of the Anthracite Coal Strike Commission, January 9, 1903, p. 4554.

It was about seven o'clock in the evening: Testimony of John Harvilla, Boiler Operator for Coxe Bros. & Co., Transcript of the Anthracite Coal Strike Commission, January 9, 1903, p. 4553.

a tip from a North Lehigh cop: Letter from E. A. Oberrender to L. C. Smith, August 27, 1902; Letter from Charles Rohland to John Rohland, September 3, 1902, Coxe Family Mining Papers, 3005, Box 561, Folder 13, HSP.

He found John Gordon giving out relief orders to striking miners: Letter from W. A. Evans to E. A. Oberrender, September 6, 1902, Coxe Family Mining Papers, 3005, Box 561, Folder 13, HSP.

***See there*, Gordon said, pointing to the house, *damn scab got shot*:** Letter from W. A. Evans to E. A. Oberrender, September 6, 1902.

don't have him arrested yet: Letter from W. A. Evans to L. C. Smith, September 23, 1902, Coxe Family Mining Papers, 3005, Box 561, Folder 23, HSP.

Some of his reports were just updates: Letter from W. A. Evans to L. C. Smith, September 23, 1902.

he was in it proper for a scheme: Letter from W. A. Evans to E. A. Oberrender, September 20, 1902, Coxe Family Mining Papers, 3005, Box 560, Folder 3, HSP.

he'd *gleaned considerable information*: Letter from W. A. Evans to L. C. Smith, September 26, 1902, Coxe Family Mining Papers, 3005, Box 560, Folder 3, HSP.

You have to understand, there's no easy road: W. A. Evans to L. C. Smith, September 28, 1902, Coxe Family Mining Papers, 3005, Box 560, Folder 3, HSP.

Smith told Oberrender to pay Evans: Oberrender's Notes, August 11, 1902, Coxe Family Mining Papers, Box 560, Folder 3, HSP.

You are hereby asked by the U.M.W. of A.: Oberrender's Notes, June 9, 1902, Coxe Family Mining Papers, Box 561, Folder 22, HSP.

only at higher rates: Testimony of Thomas McNamara, Commonwealth v. Stephen Drosdick, July 16, 1902, Coxe Family Mining Papers, 3005, Box 560, Folder 18, p. 5.

My family cannot go anywhere: Testimony of Thomas McNamara, Commonwealth v. Stephen Drosdick, July, 16 1902, p. 8.

the only name that appeared on the Oneida boycott: Letter from Oberrender to Smith, June 30, 1902, Coxe Family Mining Papers, 3005, Box 560, Folder 11, HSP.

heard some action taken: Letter from Oberrender to Smith, July 18, 1902, Coxe Family Mining Papers, Box 561, Folder 2, HSP.

if you'd have listened to me: Oberrender transcribed Kahley's and his wife's argument in handwriting at the bottom of a copy of the affidavit he brought with him, Affidavit of Frank Kahley, November 20, 1902, Coxe Family Mining Papers, Box 561, Folder 23, HSP.

I attended the meeting of the Sheppton Local of the United Mine Workers: Affidavit of Frank Kahley, November 20, 1902.

When she finished, she handed it to Kahley: Smith congratulated Oberrender on his work on the Dettrey case, telling him it might finally be "possible that an injunction may be gotten out" against the union because of it: Letter from Smith to Oberrender, November 18, 1902, Coxe Family Mining Papers, Box 561, Folder 23, HSP.

Hudock was convicted of conspiracy and jailed: Transcript of Testimony, Commonwealth v. Stephen Drosdick and Edward Malloy, July 16, 1902, Coxe Family Mining Papers, Box 560, Folder 18, HSP.

Dettrey was acquitted of the charges: Testimony of John T. Lenahan, Transcript of the Anthracite Coal Strike Commission, January 9, 1902, NARA II, Vol. 29, Box 5, p. 4,520; Testimony of W. H. Dettrey, Transcript of the Anthracite Coal Strike Commission, December 3, 1902, NARA II, Vol. 10, Box 2, p. 1142.

Oberrender kept a detailed diary of the strike: "Statement and Summary of Various Overt Acts Since the Inauguration of Strike up to Date, as Requested by Mr. John T. Lenahan," Coxe Family Mining Papers, Box 561, Folder 22, HSP.

so he'd know who to fire when the strike ended: Testimony of William E. Markwick, Engineer at D.L.&W.'s Sloane Mine, Transcript of the Anthracite Coal Strike Commission, December 5, 1902, Scranton, PA, NARA II, Vol. 12, Box 2, pp. 1407–8; "Statement and Summary of Various Overt Acts Since the Inauguration of Strike up to Date, as Requested by Mr. John T. Lenahan," Coxe Family Mining Papers, Box 561, Folder 22, HSP; Oberrender's Notes, June 9, 1902.

Chapter 5: The Occupation of Shenandoah

shut in by high hills: US Department of Labor, Children's' Bureau, Publication No. 106, Child Labor and the Welfare of Children in an Anthracite Coal-Mining District, 1922, Government Printing Office, Washington, DC, p. 1.

a curse to everything above: For a description of the mammoth vein, see the Testimony of Thomas Whildin, General Inside Foreman of Lehigh Coal

& Navigation Co., Transcript of the Anthracite Coal Strike Commission, January 28, 1903, Philadelphia, PA, NARA II, Vol. 45, Box 7, pp. 7,677–757; Victor R. Greene, *The Slavic Community on Strike: Immigrant Labor in Pennsylvania Anthracite* (Notre Dame: University of Notre Dame Press, 1968), 6.

who lived in shanty settlements: US Department of Labor, Child Labor and the Welfare of Children, p. 3.

children died of starvation than any other cause: On accidents, see Peter Roberts, *Anthracite Coal Communities: A Study of the Demography, the Social, Educational and Moral Life of the Anthracite Region* (New York: Macmillan, 1904), 78. On police violence, see Reading Company, Secretary's Office, No. 178, "Partial List of Acts of Violence or Intimidation During the Anthracite Strike of 1902," Reading Company Collection, Box 1203, Folder 3277, Hagley Library and Archive. On the health and welfare of children, see US Department of Labor, Children's Bureau, Publication No. 106, Child Labor and the Welfare of Children in an Anthracite Coal-Mining District, 1922, Government Printing Office, Washington, DC.

***polinky*-drinking Polanders and coarse and unkind *Huns*:** See Transcript of the Anthracite Coal Strike Commission; Harold W. Aurand, *Coalcracker Culture: Work and Values in Pennsylvania Anthracite, 1835–1935* (Selinsgrove: Susquehanna University Press, 2003), 76; Emily Greene Balch, *Our Slavic Fellow Citizens* (New York: Charities Publication Committee, 1910), 7; Stewart Culin, *A Trooper's Narrative of Service in the Anthracite Coal Strike*, 1902 (Philadelphia: G. W. Jacobs & co., 1903), 42.

a citizen's alliance would declare itself: "Hazleton Citizens Organize," *Miners' Journal*, July 5, 1902, p. 3.

***No Police Protection*:** See *Miners' Journal*, August 1, 4–5, 1902.

Strikers Arrested: *Miners' Journal*, August 6, 1902.

Military Rule Assures Peace: *Miners' Journal*, August 7, 1902.

all riots would be quelled: Shenandoah "is quieter than before the recent outbreak, and there is no doubt now that any disturbance that occurs will be crushed before assuming a dangerous or even troublesome aspect." See "Military Rule Assures Peace," *Miners' Journal*, August 7, 1902, p. 1.

***Operators Still Firm*:** See *Miners' Journal*, October 2, 3, 1902.

***J. P. Morgan Can Settle It*:** See *Miners' Journal*, October 13, 14, 16, 25, 27, 1902.

sent two machinists to Shenandoah: Testimony of George W. Good, Transcript of the Anthracite Coal Strike Commission, January 7, 1903,

Philadelphia, PA, NARA II, Vol. 27, Box 4, p. 4244.

Isn't my life *as sweet* as his?: "The First Riot Case," *Miners' Journal*, September 6, 1902.

strafing them with rifle fire: "Coroner's Jury Hears Evidence," Shenandoah *Weekly Herald*, August 9, 1902.

They made their escape: Testimony of George W. Good, Transcript of the Anthracite Coal Strike Commission, January 7, 1903, p. 4244; Report of Thomas Beddall, Deputy Sheriff, August 1, 1902, Governor William A. Stone Collection, 1898–1903, MG 181, Box 2, Folder: Executive Correspondence, 1902: Coal Strikes N.G.P. & Shenandoah Riots, Pennsylvania State Archives, Harrisburg, PA.

in a panicked, drunken rampage: Testimony of George W. Good, Transcript of the Anthracite Coal Strike Commission, January 7, 1903, pp. 4259–60.

In the version the police told: "A Busy Day on the Hill," *Miners' Journal*, September 4, 1902.

Uncle Dan beat the wooden-legged man: Uncle Dan's real name was Anthony Kauliewicz, "The Coroner's Inquest," *Miners' Journal*, August 8, 1902.

others swore it was a clothes prop: "Mob's Victim Died Late Last Evening," *Miners' Journal*, August 1, 1902; "Another Arrest; For Murder," Shenandoah *Weekly Herald*, August 9, 1902.

***caused the gun to explode*:** "Korkosky Tells How Paliewicz was Seen by Him Beating Beddall," *Shenandoah Weekly Herald*, November 15, 1902, p. 1; "Coroner Holds Inquest," *Miners' Journal*, August 8, 1902.

fifty dollars for *swearing against Paliewicz*: "Korkosky Tells How Paliewicz was Seen by Him Beating Beddall," Shenandoah *Weekly Herald*, November 15, 1902, p. 1.

it was just a witness fee: "Commonwealth Rested and Asked First Degree Verdict," Shenandoah *Weekly Herald*, November 15, 1902.

arrested a breaker boy: "Not Guilty of Beddall Murder," *Shenandoah Evening Herald*, November 21, 1902, p. 1.

Two striking miners bled to death: "Doctors Kept Busy," *Miners' Journal*, August 1, 1902.

John P. S. Gobin rode into Shenandoah: Testimony of John P. S. Gobin, Brigadier General of N.P.S. & Lt. Gov. of PA, Transcript of the Anthracite Coal Strike Commission, January 9, 1902, Philadelphia, PA, NARA II, Vol. 29, Box 5, p. 4578.

The backbone of the strike: "Their Opinion," *Miners' Journal*, August 1, 1902.

For his headquarters, he took the Ferguson Hotel: "Quiet and Order Now Prevails," Shenandoah *Weekly Herald*, August 2, 1902.

***They must depend on me to keep order*:** Testimony of John P. S. Gobin, Brigadier General of N.P.S. & Lt. Gov. of PA, Transcript of the Anthracite Coal Strike Commission, January 9, 1902, p. 4583.

***Tomahawk rights*:** Tomahawk rights refer to the patent to land acquired as an official reward for fighting Native peoples. Justices of the peace confirmed patents to land claims to all those who could prove they fought for it, whether they won or not. See Norman B. Wilkinson, "Land Policy and Speculation in Pennsylvania, 1779–1880" (PhD diss., University of Pennsylvania, 1958), 98, 222.

the Civil War interrupted his plans: "Commander of the Third Brigade," *Lebanon Daily News*, July 25, 1885; "Slate Notes," *Elk County Advocate*, September 27, 1877; "Events of the Great War for Wages," *Reading Daily Eagle*, July 25, 1877.

brigadier general in 1885: "The Lebanon Leader," Philadelphia *Times*, March 24, 1890.

a military reserve at Mt. Gretna: "What is Doing in Coalfields," *Miners' Journal*, August 12, 1902; "Camp Notes," Shenandoah *Weekly Herald*, September 13, 1902, p. 4.

***in every strike in the anthracite region*:** Testimony of John P. S. Gobin, Brigadier General of N.P.S. & Lt. Gov. of PA, Transcript of the Anthracite Coal Strike Commission, January 9, 1902, p. 4640.

he hunted the Mollies by horseback: Testimony of John P. S. Gobin, Brigadier General of N.P.S. & Lt. Gov. of PA, Transcript of the Anthracite Coal Strike Commission, January 9, 1902, p. 4641; Kevin Kenney, *Making Sense of the Molly Maguires* (Oxford: Oxford University Press, 1998), 109; Harold Aurand, *From the Molly Maguires to the United Mine Workers: The Social Ecology of an Industrial Union, 1869–1897* (Philadelphia: Temple University Press, 1971), 88–92; "The Lebanon Leader," *Philadelphia Times*, March 24, 1890, p. 3.

infantry traded fire with strikers in Jeddo: "Forward! March!" *Philadelphia Inquirer*, April 8, 1875; "Miners' Strike," *Philadelphia Inquirer*, April 10, 1875.

headquarters in the Lehigh Valley Coal Company offices: "Twenty-one Dead; Five are Dying," *Philadelphia Inquirer*, September 21, 1897.

he occupied Shenandoah: "Rushing Response of State's Guard to Call to Arms," *Philadelphia Inquirer*, September 23, 1900.

While strikers watched from the high ground: See Culin, *A Trooper's*

Narrative; Testimony of John P. S. Gobin, Brigadier General of N.P.S. & Lt. Gov. of PA, Transcript of the Anthracite Coal Strike Commission, January 9, 1902, p. 4630.

The way they jump on and off the freight trains: Testimony of John P. S. Gobin, Brigadier General of N.P.S. & Lt. Gov. of PA, Transcript of the Anthracite Coal Strike Commission, January 9, 1902, p. 4684.

in preparation to attack the soldiers: "Go Away From Home to Learn Strike News," *Shenandoah Weekly Herald*, August 9, 1902.

he sent small details of soldiers into the mine patches: Testimony of John P. S. Gobin, Brigadier General of N.P.S. & Lt. Gov. of PA, Transcript of the Anthracite Coal Strike Commission, January 9, 1902, p. 4607.

their faces blackened with coal dust: Culin, *A Trooper's Narrative*, 26.

polite boys and girls wandered into camp: Culin, *A Trooper's Narrative*, 30–32.

Maybe it'll keep the man from disturbing us again: Testimony of John P. S. Gobin, Brigadier General of N.P.S. & Lt. Gov. of PA, Transcript of the Anthracite Coal Strike Commission, January 9, 1902, p. 4590.

a club for capitalists and monopolists: "Letter to Mitchell," *Miners' Journal*, August 2, 1902; "Mitchell Replies," *Shenandoah Weekly Herald*, August 2, 1902.

It is the history of past coal strikes: "Their Opinion," *Miners' Journal*, August 1, 1902.

ignore the operators' claims of poverty: "The President Takes a Hand," *Miners' Journal*, August 14, 1902.

but the governor refused: "Governor Stone Replies," *Miners' Journal*, August 4, 1902.

Gobin spent his days talking to coal superintendents: Testimony of Richard Beamish, Reporter for *The North American*, Transcript of the Coal Strike Commission, January 12, 1903, Philadelphia, PA, NARA II, Vol. 31, Box 5, pp. 5010–11; See also, "Military Rule Assures Peace," *Miners' Journal*, August 7, 1902; "Another Arrest" and "Thirty-One Warrants," *Miners' Journal*, August 11, 1902.

Scab! Vile dog! Government hobo!: "Lansford and Summit Hill," *Miners' Journal*, August 28, 1902.

schoolteacher niece Anna, sister to the murdered Joseph Beddall: "Affected the Teachers," *Miners' Journal*, August 26, 1902.

Gobin fell asleep to the distant sound of dynamite: "After that they began to dynamite around my own headquarters. It got to be really very uncomfortably close. I would hear one or two explosions at night." Testimony of John P. S. Gobin, Brigadier General of N.P.S. & Lt. Gov. of PA, Transcript of the Anthracite Coal Strike Commission, January 9, 1902, p. 4619.

***I fear there will be more trouble in the morning*:** Testimony of John P. S. Gobin, Brigadier General of N.P.S. & Lt. Gov. of PA, Transcript of the Anthracite Coal Strike Commission, January 9, 1902, p. 4599; "Sharp Shooting," *Miners' Journal*, August 20, 1902.

***a secret movement*:** "I made a secret movement. I wanted to get there during the night and I took a battalion of the 12th Regiment, got them on the cars and with myself left Shenandoah at midnight. I reached there about four o'clock in the morning before daylight. I moved my troops quietly up into what was represented to me—I met a deputy sheriff—the deputy sheriff met me as I reached there. I went with him up into the upper region of Lansford and found a baseball park where I could let my men get some breakfast. We slept in the baseball park until morning. As quick as it began to get daylight, however, the crowds began to assemble all around." Testimony of P. S. Gobin, Brigadier General of N.P.S. & Lt. Gov. of PA, Transcript of the Anthracite Coal Strike Commission, January 9, 1902, Philadelphia, PA, NARA II, Vol. 29, Box 5, p. 4590.

***all the acts of violence*:** "Quiet at Nesquehoning," *Miners' Journal*, August 20, 1902.

***I'll give you one too*:** "The Deputies are Held," *Miners' Journal*, August 25, 1902.

***He was shot down like a dog*:** "Sharpe was Martyr," *Miners' Journal*, August 22, 1902.

***Men were assaulted*:** Testimony of John P. S. Gobin, Brigadier General of N.P.S. & Lt. Gov. of PA, Transcript of the Anthracite Coal Strike Commission, January 9, 1902, p. 4607.

troops weren't reliable: "Bands Hard to Get, and Drum Corps May Enlist," Shenandoah *Weekly Herald*, September 20, 1902.

We need federal troops: "Operators Want Federal Troops," *Philadelphia Inquirer*, October 9, 1902.

A Pottsville paper estimated: "What is Doing in Coalfields," *Miners' Journal*, August 12, 1902.

an entire company of troops raised a cheer to John Mitchell: "Gobin Day at Duryea," *Miners' Journal*, September 26, 1902.

***should have called up the Philadelphia regiments first*:** Testimony of John P. S. Gobin, Brigadier General of N.P.S. & Lt. Gov. of PA, Transcript of the Anthracite Coal Strike Commission, January 9, 1902, p. 4592. See also "Camp Notes," *Shenandoah Weekly Herald*, August 30, 1902.

Gobin sent two battalions to Tamaqua and Lansford: "Lansford and Summit Hill," *Miners' Journal*, August 28, 1902.

use your bayonets if at all possible: "Headquarters Third Brigade, N.G.P., Shenandoah, PA, August 29, 1902, General Orders No. 3", Testimony of John P. S. Gobin, Brigadier General of N.P.S. & Lt. Gov. of PA, Transcript of the Anthracite Coal Strike Commission, January 9, 1902, pp. 4625–26.

a wise course to pursue: "Arbitration Bill," *Miners' Journal*, September 1, 1902, p. 2.

issued ball cartridges for their carbines: Testimony of John P. S. Gobin, Brigadier General of N.P.S. & Lt. Gov. of PA, Transcript of the Anthracite Coal Strike Commission, January 9, 1902, p. 4625.

The harboring of disorderly persons: "Col. Clement Determined," *Miners' Journal*, September 26, 1902, p. 2.

and burned the place to the ground: "Upset the Lamp," *Miners' Journal*, September 9, 1902.

it must have been a meteor that did it: "Dynamited his House," *Miners' Journal*, September 25, 1902.

It must have been cut to pieces and hauled away: "Troops May be Sent," *Miners' Journal*, September 9, 1902.

guarding the coal trains that came out of the washeries: Though Gobin claimed the use of troops to escort scabs was not a regular practice, it was the one tactic used in every military strikebreaking occupation. See Robert V. Bruce, *1877, Year of Violence* (Chicago: Ivan R. Dee Publisher, 1989), 18, 67; Grace Palladino, *Another Civil War: Labor, Capital, and the State in the Anthracite Regions of Pennsylvania, 1840–68* (Champaign: University of Illinois Press, 1990), 144–46; Matthew Margis, "America's Progressive Army: How the National Guard Grew out of Progressive Era Reforms" (PhD diss., Iowa State University, 2016), 64, 76; Joseph John Holmes, "The National Guard of Pennsylvania: Policemen or Industry, 1865–1905" (PhD diss., University of Connecticut, 1971).

after the governor sent the Second City Troop of Philadelphia: "Soldiers Make Uneventful Trip," *Miners' Journal*, September 2, 1902.

selling asbestos coal bricks soaked in oil: Cornell, *The Anthracite Coal Strike of 1902*, 174, note 5.

They were shocked to find no takers: "Looking for Miners," Shenandoah *Weekly Herald*, September 27, 1902.

donated more than a thousand dollars: "Business Men's Association Getting Ready to Spread Money," Shenandoah *Weekly Herald*, September 13, 1902.

Doctors began treating strikers: "Notice to the Mine Workers," Shenandoah *Weekly Herald*, September 13, 1902.

The UMW opened five stores in Shamokin: "Shamokin Mine Workers Open Several Relief Stores," Shenandoah *Weekly Herald*, September 20, 1902.

could take care of the strikers indefinitely: "Treasurer Wilson Hopeful," Shenandoah *Weekly Herald*, September 13, 1902.

voted unanimously to remain out of work: "Wm. Penn's Three Local Unions Adopt Resolution of Loyalty," Shenandoah *Weekly Herald*, September 13, 1902; "Lost Creek Union Men Firm," Shenandoah *Weekly Herald*, September 13, 1902.

killing a soldier in late September: "The Twelfth Suffering," Shenandoah *Weekly Herald*, September 20, 1902.

refused to serve in the occupation: "Bands Hard to Get, and Drum Corps May Enlist," Shenandoah *Weekly Herald*, September 20, 1902.

Troopers began sharing their rations: Testimony of Father Patrick McMahon, Minersville Priest, Transcript of the Anthracite Coal Strike Commission, February 3, 1903, Philadelphia, PA, NARA II, Vol. 49, Box 8, p. 8639.

but only if they quit immediately: "The Soldiers and Strikers," *Miners' Journal*, October 11, 1902.

toddlers went from house to house yelling scab: "They Make Complaint," *Miners' Journal*, September 12, 1902.

to the White House for a meeting: See Cornell, *The Anthracite Coal Strike of 1902*, 179.

***the strike cannot be broken*:** "Mr. Mitchell Makes Answer," *Miners' Journal*, October 9, 1902.

The only thing left to do was to send in the entire national guard, which the governor did in early October: "Mob at Plymouth," *Miners' Journal*, October 2, 1902.

Gobin sent field artillery: "Troops Will Arrive Today," *Miners' Journal*, October 8, 1902.

All units had Gatling guns: "Guardsmen are with Us," *Miners' Journal*, October 9, 1902.

Nearly two thousand strikers: "At Mt. Carmel," *Miners' Journal*, October 1, 1902.

brought field artillery to Shenandoah: "Second Brigade," *Miners' Journal*,

October 9, 1902.

weren't many nonunion men left to protect: "Second Brigade," *Miners' Journal*, October 9, 1902.

and sent in the troops: "Mitchell Calls up Platt," *Miners' Journal*, October 11, 1902.

they could not force the men back to work: "Mr. Mitchell Makes Answer," *Miners' Journal*, October 9, 1902.

secret meetings in a yacht: "No Meeting Tomorrow," *Miners' Journal*, October 13, 1902.

George Baer start ducking into side doors: "The Coal Presidents," *Miners' Journal*, October 14, 1902.

friendly to organized labor: "Will Investigate the Roads," *Miners' Journal*, October 20, 1902.

Chapter 6: The Jeddo Evictions

***dictator of the coal business*:** as quoted in Robert J. Cornell, *The Anthracite Coal Strike of 1902* (New York: Russell & Russell, 1971), 127.

We will not surrender: Quoted in Cornell, The *Anthracite Coal Strike of 1902*, 115.

***could not appear on record as President of the United Mine Workers*:** Testimony of George Baer, Transcript of the Anthracite Coal Strike Commission, October 27, 1902, Scranton, PA, NARA II, Vol. 1, Box 1, p. 8.

When the deal went public: Cornell, *The Anthracite Coal Strike of 1902*, 234.

***They know they're beaten*:** Mary Harris Jones, The *Autobiography of Mother Jones* (Chicago: Charles H. Kerr Publishing Co., 1925), 62.

I am informed through intermediaries: "The Morning Session," *Miners' Journal*, October 21, 1902.

We recognize the right of capital to consolidate: "The Morning Session."

***Some might not get their old places back*:** "Convention Adjourns Until this Morning," *Miners' Journal*, October 21, 1902.

***I earnestly hope and firmly believe*:** "Mitchell Pleased," *Wilkes-Barre Times Leader*, October 21, 1902.

***All men desiring to work for us*:** Testimony of Sidney Williams, General Superintendent of G. B. Markle & Co., Transcript of the Anthracite Coal Strike Commission, January 26, 1903, Scranton, PA, NARA II, Vol. 43, Box 7, pp. 7347–48.

What's your age?: Testimony of Sidney Williams, Transcript of the Anthracite Coal Strike Commission, January 26, 1903, p. 7351.

Criminal acts: Testimony of Charlie Helferty, Transcript of the Anthracite Coal Strike Commission, December 8, 1902, Scranton, PA, NARA II, Vol. 14, Box 3, p. 1858.

you licked some parties in Freeland: Testimony of Gottleib Filler, Transcript of the Anthracite Coal Strike Commission, January 26, 1903, Philadelphia, PA, NARA II, Vol. 43, Box 7, p. 7404.

You'll never work for the company again: Testimony of Paul Dunleavy, Transcript of the Anthracite Coal Strike Commission, December 8, 1902, Philadelphia, PA, NARA II, Vol. 14, Box 3, 1745.

Could I at least get a recommendation so I can find another job?: Testimony of Frank Ray, Transcript of the Anthracite Coal Strike Commission, December 8, 1902, Philadelphia, PA, NARA II, Vol. 14, Box 3, p. 1736.

All were turned away: On the use of the coal companies' use of the blacklist, see Testimony of John Mitchell, President of the United Mine Workers of America, Transcript of the Anthracite Coal Strike Commission, November 18, 1902, Scranton, PA, NARA II, Vol. 5, Box 1, p. 555: "The blacklist is the more baneful [than the boycott]. I do not know whether the blacklist is used now in the Anthracite fields but many of the miners believe it has been and believe it is. If a man loses his job in one mine he may hunt and hunt all over the Anthracite region for another job and be unable to get one, without any reasons being assigned by those from whom he seeks employment"; When asked why union membership lists were not made public, George Hartlein, secretary, UMW District 9, said, "It became necessary to insert that into the obligation of labor organizations, to prevent a man, if possible, from telling an employer the name of another man who was a member of the Organization. While we have no specific information that the men have been directly discharged for belonging to a labor organization, yet men being employed at a colliery for years, and no objection found to them, as soon as they became members of a labor organization it seemed that there was no work for them one way or another, and we took it for granted, that was the reason." Testimony of George Hartlein, Secretary of UMW District 9, Transcript of the Anthracite Coal Strike Commission, February 5, 1903, Philadelphia, PA, NARA II, Vol. 51, Box 9, p. 9105; See also Victor R. Greene, *The Slavic Community on Strike: Immigrant Labor in Pennsylvania Anthracite* (Notre Dame: University of Notre Dame Press, 1968); On the use of blacklists in the western Pennsylvania bituminous coalfields, see Letter from A. W. Calloway, Florence Mine Supt. To Lucius Robinson, President of the Rochester & Pittsburgh Coal & Iron Company, July 7, 1902, Rochester & Pittsburgh Coal Company Records, MG 51, Box

1, Folder 7, Early Executive Correspondence Letter Book, Indiana University of Pennsylvania Special Collections and Archives, Indiana, PA.

As a condition precedent to my employment at A. Pardee & Co.: "Misunderstand Agreement and Hesitate to Sign," *Hazleton Sentinel*, October 23, 1902.

picketed all the roads that led to Markle's collieries: Testimony of Sidney Williams, Transcript of the Anthracite Coal Strike Commission, January 26, 1903, p. 7323.

***to personally consider these men's cases*:** Testimony of Sidney Williams, Transcript of the Anthracite Coal Strike Commission, January 26, 1903, p. 7328.

***There are certain men who can never return*:** Testimony of Sidney Williams, Transcript of the Anthracite Coal Strike Commission, January 26, 1903, p. 7354.

***It might expose certain men to the revenge*:** Comment of Samuel Dickson, Attorney for G. B. Markle & Sons, during the testimony of Sidney Williams, Transcript of the Anthracite Coal Strike Commission, January 26, 1903, p. 7327.

***There never was a victory yet*:** Testimony of James Gallagher, Transcript of the Anthracite Coal Strike Commission, December 6, 1902, Scranton, PA, NARA II, Vol. 13, Box 3, p. 1652.

***We go back in a body or not at all*:** Telegram from George Markle to Carroll Wright, October 25, 1902, in Testimony of Sidney Williams, Transcript of the Anthracite Coal Strike Commission, January 26, 1903, p. 7245.

***Our men have not returned to work*:** Telegram from Markle to Wright, quoted in the testimony of Sidney Williams, Transcript of the Anthracite Coal Strike Commission, January 26, 1903, pp. 7354–57.

***since I came to the country*:** Testimony of James Gallagher, Transcript of the Anthracite Coal Strike Commission, December 6, 1902, p. 1673.

***It's not permitted*:** Testimony of Daniel J. McCarthy, Transcript of the Anthracite Coal Strike Commission, January 26, 1903, Scranton, PA, NARA II, Vol. 43, Box 7, p. 7229.

These are *cut-throat agreements*: Testimony of Daniel J. McCarthy, Transcript of the Anthracite Coal Strike Commission, January 26, 1903, Philadelphia, PA, NARA II, Vol. 43, Box 7, p. 7215.

***I'm in sympathy with these men*:** Testimony of Daniel J. McCarthy, Transcript of the Anthracite Coal Strike Commission, January 26, 1903, Philadelphia, PA, NARA II, Vol. 43, Box 7, p. 7215.

the sheriff marched into Jeddo: "Pathetic Scenes Attend Evictions," *Philadelphia Inquirer*, November 7, 1902; "The Markle Evictions," *Wilkes-Barre Daily News*, November 7, 1902.

***What could I do?*:** Testimony of Daniel J. McCarthy, Transcript of the Anthracite Coal Strike Commission, January 26, 1903, Philadelphia, PA, NARA II, Vol. 43, Box 7, p. 7,216.

They were small villages of wood-framed structures: Peter Roberts, *Anthracite Coal Communities: A Study of the Demography, the Social, Educational and Moral Life of the Anthracite Region* (New York: Macmillan, 1904), 128.

The Philadelphia and Reading Coal and Iron Co. rented 2,000 shanties: Testimony of KC Wilson, Transcript of the Anthracite Coal Strike Commission, February 2, 1903, Philadelphia, PA, NARA II, Vol. 48, Box 8, p. 8258.

The Lehigh Coal Co. rented out 700: Testimony of James McCready, Transcript of the Anthracite Coal Strike Commission, January 28, 1903, Scranton, PA, NARA II, Vol. 45, Box 7, p. 7778.

Coxe Bros. & Co. rented out 879. Van Wickle leased 300: Roberts, *Anthracite Coal Communities*, 128.

Markle rented more than 500 shanties for fifteen cents a day: Testimony of Sidney Williams, Transcript of the Anthracite Coal Strike Commission, January 26, 1903, p. 7330; Statement of Clarence Darrow, Lawyer for the United Mine Workers, Transcript of the Anthracite Coal Strike Commission, January 26, 1903, Philadelphia, PA, NARA II, Vol. 43, Box 7, p. 7242; Roberts, *Anthracite Coal Communities*, 128.

He suffered constant headaches from when a roof fell: Arrested: *Hazleton Sentinel*, May 25, 1896; both legs broken: Hazleton *Daily Standard*, August 16, 1893; crushed nearly to death: Hazleton *Plain Speaker*, January 12, 1899.

***sick and blind besides*:** Testimony of Henry Coll, Testimony of James McCready, Transcript of the Anthracite Coal Strike Commission, December 9, 1902, Scranton, PA, NARA II, Vol. 15, Box 3, p. 1900.

***You got a six-days' notice*:** Henry Coll Testimony, Transcript of the Anthracite Coal Strike Commission, December 9, 1902, Scranton, PA, NARA II, Vol. 15, Box 3, p. 1909.

***You had ample time*:** Testimony of Sidney Williams, Transcript of the Anthracite Coal Strike Commission, January 26, 1903, p. 7336.

***cannot have five minutes now*:** Henry Coll had more than one son. He knew he "was doomed" when his oldest son became president of the local union. "Where is your son now?" asked Darrow. "He is in retreat; he is on the other side of Wilkes-Barre. He got a little melancholy and so he is now in the hospital." Testimony of Henry Coll, Testimony of James McCready, Transcript of the Anthracite Coal Strike Commission, December 9, 1902, Scranton, PA, NARA II, Vol. 15, Box 3, pp. 1906–7.

This is very sudden, ain't it?: Testimony of Paul Dunleavy, Jeddo Miner for G. B. Markle & Co., Transcript of the Anthracite Coal Strike Commission, December 8, 1902, Scranton, PA, NARA II, Vol. 14, Box 3, p. 1747.

The cops were working quickly now: "G. B. Markle & Co. Evict Tenants," *Pottsville Republican*, November 7, 1902.

Good morning, Henry: Testimony of Henry Shovlin, Transcript of the Anthracite Coal Strike Commission, December 9, 1902, Scranton, PA, NARA II, Vol. 14, Box 3, p. 1777.

sixty bushels of potatoes: Testimony of Sidney Williams, Transcript of the Anthracite Coal Strike Commission, January 26, 1903, p. 7335.

seven barrels of sauerkraut: Testimony of Sidney Williams, Transcript of the Anthracite Coal Strike Commission, January 26, 1903, p. 7335.

They called Gallagher *Granny*: Testimony of James Gallagher, Transcript of the Anthracite Coal Strike Commission, December 6, 1902, p. 1655.

hadn't been paid in nearly eighteen years: Darrow: "How long did you work at that place without drawing any money?" Gallagher: "About seventeen years and nine months. (Laughter)": Testimony of James Gallagher, Transcript of the Anthracite Coal Strike Commission, December 6, 1902, p. 1635.

Mr. Markle, what did you throw me out for?: Testimony of James Gallagher, Transcript of the Anthracite Coal Strike Commission, February 5, 1903, Philadelphia, PA, NARA II, Vol. 51, Box 9, p. 9011.

Why didn't you move out when the time was up to move: Testimony of Andrew Hannik, Transcript of the Anthracite Coal Strike Commission, December 9, 1902, Scranton, PA, NARA II, Vol. 15, Box 3, p. 1892.

go to Paul Dunleavy's and get help: Testimony of Henry Coll, Transcript of the Anthracite Coal Strike Commission, December 9, 1902, Scranton, PA, NARA II, Vol. 15, Box 3, p. 1914.

You people was evicted: Testimony of Henry Coll, Transcript of the Anthracite Coal Strike Commission, December 9, 1902, Scranton, PA, NARA II, Vol. 15, Box 3, p. 1915.

***lay down at half-past* ten to go to sleep:** Testimony of Henry Coll, Transcript of the Anthracite Coal Strike Commission, December 9, 1902, Scranton, PA, NARA II, Vol. 15, Box 3, p. 1916.

Chapter 7: Show Us the Lung of a Miner

is by the strong arm of the military at your command: As quoted in Robert J. Cornell, *The Anthracite Coal Strike of 1902* (New York: Russell & Russell, 1971), 185.

***This is an investigation by a commission*:** Comment of E. B. Thomas, Chairman of the Board of Pennsylvania Coal and Hillside Coal and Iron Co., Transcript of the Anthracite Coal Strike Commission, October 27 1902, Washington, D.C., NARA II, Vol. 1, Box 1, p. 11.

It's a concession to humanity: Cornell, *The Anthracite Coal Strike of 1902*, 222.

Roosevelt puts a military man on the commission: See Cornell, *The Anthracite Coal Strike of 1902*, 230–31, note 60.

We're in favor of taking back the old employees: "Commission in Lehigh Region," *Hazleton Sentinel*, November 3, 1902.

husbands and fathers are still alive: "Commission in Lehigh Region," *Hazleton Sentinel*, November 3, 1902.

***works his way up, step by step*:** Testimony of John Mitchell, President of the United Mine Workers of America, November 14, 1902, Transcript of the Anthracite Coal Strike Commission, Scranton, PA, NARA II, Vol. 2, Box 1, pp. 9–29.

tells harrowing stories of dangerous working conditions: Testimony of Mike Midlick, Miner at Eckley for Coxe Bros. & Co., Transcript of the Anthracite Coal Strike Commission, December 3, 1902, Scranton, PA, NARA II, Vol. 10, Box 2, p. 1,205; Testimony of Peter G. Gallagher, Miner for G. B. Markle & Co., Transcript of the Anthracite Coal Strike Commission, December 9, 1902, Scranton, PA, NARA II, Vol. 15, Box 3, p. 1927.

Darrow puts children on the stand: Testimony of James Moore, Methodist Minister from Avoca, Transcript of the Anthracite Coal Strike Commission, December 5, 1902, Scranton, PA, NARA II, Vol. 12, Box 2, pp. 1472–73; Victor R. Greene, *The Slavic Community on Strike: Immigrant Labor in Pennsylvania Anthracite* (Notre Dame: University of Notre Dame Press, 1968), 50; Harold W. Aurand, *Coalcracker Culture: Work and Values in Pennsylvania Anthracite, 1835–1935* (Selinsgrove: Susquehanna University Press, 2003), 177; Testimony of David F. Evans, Foreman at West Pittson for Stevens Coal Co., Transcript of the Anthracite Coal Strike Commission, January 23, 1903, Philadelphia, PA, NARA II, Vol. 41, Box 6, pp. 6962.

Hands mangled by machinery, bodies crushed by gears: Aurand, *Coalcracker Culture*, 177.

by fathers who need candles kept lit: Testimony of David F. Evans, Foreman at West Pittston for Stevens Coal Co., Transcript of the Anthracite Coal Strike Commission, January 23, 1903, Philadelphia, PA, NARA II, Vol. 41, Box 6, p. 6941.

Seventeen-year-old Mike Baker: Testimony of Mike Baker, Miner at Oakdale No. 4 of G. B. Markle & Co., Transcript of the Anthracite Coal Strike Commission, December 9, 1902, Scranton, PA, NARA II, Vol. 15, Box 3, pp. 1976–77.

***clubbed by the slate picker boss*:** Testimony of Mike Baker, Miner at Oakdale No. 4 of G. B. Markle & Co., Transcript of the Anthracite Coal Strike Commission, December 9, 1902, 1977–78.

***I don't get no money*:** Testimony of Andrew Chippie, Twelve-Year-Old Breaker Boy, Transcript of the Anthracite Coal Strike Commission, December 6, 1902, Scranton, PA, NARA II, Vol. 13, Box 3, pp. 1626–28.

***through the coalfield, an old custom kept up*:** Testimony of Charles C. Rose, Superintendent of Delaware & Hudson, Transcript of the Anthracite Coal Strike Commission, January 10, 1903, Philadelphia, PA, NARA II, Vol. 30, Box 5, p. 4784.

It just isn't *feasible* to abolish child labor: Testimony of W. A. May, President of Scranton Board of Trade & G. M. of Hillside/Penn Coal Co., Transcript of the Anthracite Coal Strike Commission, January 13, 1903, Philadelphia, PA, NARA II, Vol. 32, Box 5, p. 5247.

The contractors hire inexperienced mine laborers: Testimony of Henry Carver, Contractor, Transcript of the Anthracite Coal Strike Commission, February 3, 1903, Philadelphia , PA, NARA II, Vol. 49, Box 8, pp. 8547–48; Testimony of William Zorn, Contract Mine for Dunmore, Transcript of the Anthracite Coal Strike Commission, January 15, 1903, Philadelphia , PA, NARA II, Vol. 34, Box 6, p. 5639.

how Markle controls the labor process: Testimony of George O. Thomas, Inside Foreman for Clear Spring Coal Co., Transcript of the Anthracite Coal Strike Commission, January 23, 1903, Philadelphia, PA, NARA II, Vol. 41, Box 6, pp. 6918.

Most miners conserve their powder: Testimony of Henry Shovlin, Transcript of the Anthracite Coal Strike Commission, December 8, 1902, Scranton, PA, NARA II, Vol. 14, Box 3, pp. 1797–98.

Darrow asks the miners to describe their working conditions: Testimony of James Gallagher, Miner for G. B. Markle & Co., Transcript of the Anthracite Coal Strike Commission, December 6, 1902, Scranton, PA, NARA II, Vol. 13, Box 3, p. 1639.

***flying from the pick-point*:** Testimony of David E. Jones, Inside Foreman for

Lehigh Coal & Navigation Co., Transcript of the Anthracite Coal Strike Commission, January 28, 1903, Philadelphia, PA, NARA II, Vol. 45, Box 7, p. 7794.

all cut and disfigured: Testimony of Dr. Eugene J. Butler, Physician for the Poor Board of the Central Poor District of Luzerne County, Transcript of the Anthracite Coal Strike Commission, November 21, 1902, Scranton, PA, NARA II, Vol. 8, Box 2, p. 990.

Miners who have *all become anemic*: Testimony of Dr. F. P. Lenahan, Wilkes-Barre Physician, Transcript of the Anthracite Coal Strike Commission, November 20, 1902, Scranton, PA, NARA II, Vol. 7, Box 2, p. 942; Testimony of Dr. Richard Gibbons, Scranton Physician, Transcript of the Anthracite Coal Strike Commission, November 20, 1902, Scranton, PA, NARA II, NARA II, Vol. 7, Box 2, p. 961.

a chunk of anthracite coal: Testimony of Dr. F. P. Lenahan, Wilkes-Barre Physician, Transcript of the Anthracite Coal Strike Commission, November 20, 1902, Scranton, PA, NARA II, Vol. 7, Box 2, pp. 911–12.

the hospitals don't have enough beds to treat chronic cases: Testimony of Dr. F. P. Lenahan, Wilkes-Barre Physician, Transcript of the Anthracite Coal Strike Commission, November 20, 1902, Scranton, PA, NARA II, Vol. 7, Box 2, p. 941.

where he dies from causes so numerous no doctor is certain what killed him: I base this description on the thousands of hours of testimony the miners gave to the Anthracite Coal Strike Commission. See Record Group 257: Records of the Bureau of Labor Statistics; Records of the Commerce and Labor, "Transcripts of Proceedings of the Anthracite Coal Strike Commission, 1902–03," National Archives and Records Administration II, College Park, MD.

Have you here with you any samples?: Clarence Darrow question to Dr. Coplin, Testimony of Dr. W. M. L. Coplin, Professor of Pathology at Jefferson Medical College, Transcript of the Anthracite Coal Strike Commission, February 5, 1903, Philadelphia, PA, NARA II, Vol. 51, Box 9, pp. 9058–65.

***I have*, the doctor replies:** Testimony of Dr. Eugene J. Butler, Luzerne County Poor House Director, Transcript of the Anthracite Coal Strike Commission, November 21, 1902, Scranton, PA, NARA II, Vol. 8, Box 2, p. 988.

rob him of breath and eventually asphyxiate him: Testimony of Dr. O'Malley, Scranton Doctor, Transcript of the Anthracite Coal Strike Commission, November 20, 1902, Scranton, PA, NARA II, Vol. 7, Box 2, pp. 910–16.

Parts of them will: Coal Company lawyer Warren question to Dr. Coplin, Testimony of Dr. W. M. L. Coplin, Professor of Pathology at Jefferson

Medical College, Transcript of the Anthracite Coal Strike Commission, February 5, 1903, p. 9,065.

the lungs of colored men. No, sir, I think not: exchange between Bishop Spalding and Dr. Coplin, Testimony of Dr. W. M. L. Coplin, Professor of Pathology at Jefferson Medical College, Transcript of the Anthracite Coal Strike Commission, February 5, 1903, p. 9,059.

so little special training or skill: Opening Statement of James H. Torrey Esq., Lawyer for The Delaware & Hudson Company, Transcript of the Anthracite Coal Strike Commission, January 10, 1903, Philadelphia, PA, NARA II, Vol. 30, Box 5, p. 4,713.

I was working two miners and two laborers: Testimony of Daniel Evans, Contract Miner at Woodward Colliery, Transcript of the Anthracite Coal Strike Commission, February 4, 1903, Philadelphia, PA, NARA II, Vol. 50, Box 9, p. 8,766.

Divided it between him and I: Testimony of Shadrach Lewis, Contract Miner at Woodward Colliery, Transcript of the Anthracite Coal Strike Commission, February 4, 1903, Philadelphia, PA, NARA II, Vol. 50, Box 9, p. 8784.

after the colliery *deducted all expenses*: Testimony of Frank Richards, Contract Miner at Woodward Colliery, Transcript of the Anthracite Coal Strike Commission, February 4, 1903, Philadelphia, PA, NARA II, Vol. 50, Box 9, p. 8806.

Is it the job of a statistician: Darrow exchange with Newcomb, Testimony of H. T. Newcomb, Statistician and Editor for *The Railway World*, Transcript of the Anthracite Coal Strike Commission, February 4, 1903, Philadelphia, PA, NARA II, Vol. 50, Box 9, p. 8705.

The Company has furnished a schedule: Darrow question to Demko, Testimony of John Demko, Miner at Gypsy Grove, Transcript of the Anthracite Coal Strike Commission, December 17, 1902, Scranton, PA, NARA, Vol. 22, Box 3, p. 3163.

My butty and me *paid the laborers*: Testimony of John Demko, Miner at Gypsy Grove, Transcript of the Anthracite Coal Strike Commission, December 17, 1902, p. 3164.

Well, gentlemens, I was in bad position: Testimony of John Demko, Miner at Gypsy Grove, Transcript of the Anthracite Coal Strike Commission, December 17, 1902, p. 3165.

Your misleading data *shake our faith*: Judge Gray's instructions, Testimony of Peter Sitclack (also written Sisscak), Miner for Pennsylvania Coal Company, Transcript of the Anthracite Coal Strike Commission, December 17, 1902, Scranton, PA, NARA II, Vol. 22, Box 3, p. 3187.

what they call *composite* miners: Testimony of Jacob P. Jones, Philadelphia & Reading Coal & Iron Paymaster, Transcript of the Anthracite Coal Strike Commission, January 30, 1903, Philadelphia, PA, NARA II, p. 8038.

These aren't *real earnings*: Darrow objection offered during, Testimony of Jacob P. Jones, Philadelphia & Reading Coal & Iron Paymaster, Transcript of the Anthracite Coal Strike Commission, January 30, 1903, p. 8045.

***Like averaging the total earnings*:** Darrow comment during, Testimony of Jacob P. Jones, Philadelphia & Reading Coal & Iron Paymaster, Transcript of the Anthracite Coal Strike Commission, January 30, 1903, Philadelphia, PA, NARA II, Vol. 47, Box 8, pp. 8071–72.

it's not like the job requires *skill* or *intelligence*: Statement of H. C. Reynolds, Attorney Representing the Individual Operators, Transcript of the Anthracite Coal Strike Commission, January 22, 1903, Philadelphia, PA, NARA II, Vol. 40, Box 6, p. 6826.

They *seem wedded to the place*: Comment of Simon Wolverton, Attorney for Coxe Bros. & Co, during, Testimony of H. T. Newcomb, Statistician and Editor of *The Railway World*, Transcript of the Anthracite Coal Strike Commission, February 4, 1903, Philadelphia, PA, NARA II, Vol. 50, Box 9, p. 8763; Testimony of Charles C. Rose, Former Superintendent for The Delaware & Hudson Company, Transcript of the Anthracite Coal Strike Commission, January 10, 1903, Philadelphia, PA, NARA II, Vol. 30, Box 5, p. 4784.

the union holds them back: Our testimony and evidence "will utterly refute the charges that our employees are under-paid, and they will disclose when supplemented as they will be by oral testimony, that the earnings capacity of the employees is self-limited and that the men have it in their power, if their union did not interfere and hold them back, to earn much larger amounts, fully as large as, if not in excess, of the demands before the Commission." Statement of Everett Warren, Lawyer for the Hillside Coal and Iron Company and the Pennsylvania Coal Co., Transcript of the Anthracite Coal Strike Commission, January 13, 1903, Philadelphia, PA, NARA II, Vol. 32, Box 5, p. 5224.

***It's a well-known fact* they put their children to work:** Opening Statement of William Tayler, Esq., Lawyer for the St. Clair Coal Company, Transcript of the Anthracite Coal Strike Commission, January 13, 1903, Philadelphia, PA, NARA II, Vol. 46, Box 7, p. 7885.

***sit around and smoke*:** Testimony of W. A. May, General Superintendent of the Pennsylvania Coal & Iron Co., Transcript of the Anthracite Coal Strike Commission, February 5, 1903, Philadelphia, PA, NARA II, Vol. 51, Box 9, p. 8936.

Blame it on *their intemperance*: Opening Statement of H. C. Reynolds, Esq., Lawyer for the Independent Operators, Transcript of the Anthracite Coal Strike Commission, January 22, 1903, Philadelphia, PA, NARA II, Vol. 40, Box 6, p. 6840.

It's not like they're *American born*: Comment of Wayne MacVeagh, Attorney for the Penn. Coal Company and the Hillside Coal and Iron Co. Transcript of the Anthracite Coal Strike Commission, November 15, 1902, Scranton, PA, NARA II, Vol. 3, Box 1, pp. 247–49.

They lack *habits of frugality*: Testimony of John E. Lower, Assistant Purchaser for the Lehigh Coal & Navigation Co., Transcript of the Anthracite Coal Strike Commission, January 28, 1903, Philadelphia, PA, NARA II, Vol. 45, Box 7, p. 7809; Testimony of Charles C. Rose, Former Superintendent for The Delaware & Hudson Company, Transcript of the Anthracite Coal Strike Commission, January 24, 1903, Philadelphia, PA, NARA II, Vol. 31, Box 5, p. 4881.

***every house is a drinking place*:** Testimony of John P. S. Gobin, Brigadier General of N.P.S. & Lt. Gov. of PA, Transcript of the Anthracite Coal Strike Commission, January 9, 1902, Philadelphia, PA, NARA II, Vol. 29, Box 5, p. 4591.

They get drunk on payday and disappear for days on end: Testimony of C. W. Page, Outside Foreman for Dolph Coal Company, Transcript of the Anthracite Coal Strike Commission, January 24, 1903, Philadelphia, PA, NARA II, Vol. 42, Box 7, p. 7120; Testimony of Charles C. Rose, Former Superintendent for The Delaware & Hudson Company, Transcript of the Anthracite Coal Strike Commission, January 24, 1903, Philadelphia, PA, NARA II, Vol. 31, Box 5, p. 4881.

and stagger out of the mines barely alive: Testimony of Frank Ray, Miner for G. B. Markle & Co., Transcript of the Anthracite Coal Strike Commission, December 8, 1902, Scranton, PA, NARA II, Vol. 14, Box 3, p. 1732; Testimony of Peter Gallagher, Miner for G. B. Markle & Co., Transcript of the Anthracite Coal Strike Commission, December 9, 1902, Scranton, PA, NARA II, Vol. 15, Box 3, p. 1918.

***I lost it owing to powder smoke*:** Testimony of Thomas Powell, Miner for Delaware & Hudson, Transcript of the Anthracite Coal Strike Commission, December 5, 1902, Scranton, PA, NARA II, Vol. 12, Box 2, p. 1534.

we *work hard like a dog* but make nothing: Testimony of John Farrari, Miner for Pardee, Transcript of the Anthracite Coal Strike Commission, December 4, 1902, Scranton, PA, NARA II, Vol. 11, Box 2, p. 1292.

Or they send us to rob pillars: Testimony of Patrick J. Toolen, Miner for Delaware & Hudson Coal Co., Transcript of the Anthracite Coal Strike

Commission, February 5, 1903, Philadelphia, PA, NARA II, Vol. 51, Box 9, p. 8959.

one man should not have a loaf while the other has nothing: Comment of Clarence Darrow during, Testimony of R. S. Mercur, Superintendent of Lehigh Valley Coal Co., Transcript of the Anthracite Coal Strike Commission, January 22, 1903, Philadelphia, PA, NARA II, Vol. 40, Box 6, p. 6729.

I think the wages we are paying now are very reasonable: Testimony of Charles C. Rose, Former Superintendent for The Delaware & Hudson Company, Transcript of the Anthracite Coal Strike Commission, January 10, 1903, Philadelphia, PA, NARA II, Vol. 30, Box 5, p. 4738.

healthiest business in the world: Testimony of H. T. Newcomb, Statistician and Editor for *The Railway World*, Transcript of the Anthracite Coal Strike Commission, February 4, 1903, Philadelphia, PA, NARA II, Vol. 50, Box 9, p. 8690.

unqualified to teach kindergarten: Darrow comment during, Testimony of H.T. Newcomb, Statistician and Editor for *The Railway World*, Transcript of the Anthracite Coal Strike Commission, February 4 1903, Philadelphia, PA, NARA II, p. 8708.

dangerous to the congregation, but to the preacher?: Comment by Darrow during, Testimony of Newcomb, Statistician and Editor for *The Railway World*, Transcript of the Anthracite Coal Strike Commission, February 4, 1903, Philadelphia, PA, NARA II, p. 8694.

It was a body of men: Testimony of Ario Pardee Platt, Lattimer Killer, North Lehigh Cop, and Purchasing Agent for A. Pardee, Transcript of the Anthracite Coal Strike Commission, January 27, 1903, Philadelphia, PA., NARA II, Vol. 44, Box 7, p. 7504.

I think you are a pretty good sample: Exchange between Judge Gray and Platt, Testimony of Ario Pardee Platt, Lattimer Killer, North Lehigh Cop, and Purchasing Agent for A. Pardee, Transcript of the Anthracite Coal Strike Commission, January 27, 1903, p. 7492.

You were in the disturbance at Lattimer?: Testimony of Ario Pardee Platt, Lattimer Killer, North Lehigh Cop, and Purchasing Agent for A. Pardee, Transcript of the Anthracite Coal Strike Commission, January 27, 1903, pp. 7514–16.

The mob, do you mean?: Testimony of Ario Pardee Platt, Lattimer Killer, North Lehigh Cop, and Purchasing Agent for A. Pardee, Transcript of the Anthracite Coal Strike Commission, January 27, 1903, pp. 7508–10.

Lattimer has nothing to do with anything before us: Statement of Judge Gray during, Testimony of Ario Pardee Platt, Lattimer Killer, North Lehigh

Cop, and Purchasing Agent for A. Pardee, Transcript of the Anthracite Coal Strike Commission, January 27, 1903, Philadelphia, PA, NARA II, Vol. 44, Box 7, p. 7511.

Did the Flying Squadron make any arrests?: Testimony of Ario Pardee Platt, Lattimer Killer, North Lehigh Cop, and Purchasing Agent for A. Pardee, Transcript of the Anthracite Coal Strike Commission, January 27, 1903, p. 7515.

And the six men arrested at No. 6 on your property: Testimony of Ario Pardee Platt, Lattimer Killer, North Lehigh Cop, and Purchasing Agent for A. Pardee, Transcript of the Anthracite Coal Strike Commission, January 27, 1903, p. 7516.

The upshot of all this: Testimony Willard Young, Flying Squadron Captain & Black Powder Salesman, Transcript of the Anthracite Coal Strike Commission, January 27, 1903, Philadelphia, PA, NARA II, Vol. 44, Box 7, p. 7543.

most decidedly* under *a reign of terror: Testimony Willard Young, Flying Squadron Captain & Black Powder Salesman, Transcript of the Anthracite Coal Strike Commission, January 27, 1903, p. 7534.

The life of the mine workers: Anthracite Coal Strike Commission, "Report to the President on the of Anthracite Coal Strike" (Washington: Government Printing Office, 1903), 51.

the more businesslike and responsible it becomes: Anthracite Coal Strike Commission, "Report to the President on the Anthracite Coal Strike," 63.

most inviting inducements to entering into contractual relations: See Joe Gowaskie, "John Mitchell and the Anthracite Mine Workers: Leadership Conservatism and Rank-and-File Militancy," *Labor History* 27, no. 1 (1985): 54–83.

will result in great good and I am much pleased with it: "Mitchell is Silent," *Wilkes-Barre Semi-Weekly Record*, March 24, 1903.

means the recognition of the union is assured: "Mitchell is Silent."

The three-year agreement is an excellent one: "Counsel Wolverton Pleased," Hazleton *Standard-Speaker*, March 24, 1903.

The Lehigh Coal and Navigation company refuses to pay the higher wage rate: Grievance, January 3, 1906, Collection MG 109, Series 2, Subseries B, Box 1: Grievance Files, 13–930, Folder 19: Hazleton, Indiana University of Pennsylvania, Archives and Special Collections.

Markle reclassifies muledrivers and cuts their pay: Grievance, July 6, 1906, Collection MG 109, Series 2, Subseries B, Box 1: Grievance Files, 13–930,

Folder 145: New York, Indiana University of Pennsylvania, Archives and Special Collections.

fired for filing grievances: Joint Convention, Scranton, PA, June 15–16, 1903, Collection MG 109, Series 1, Subseries B, Box 1: Tri-District Convention Proceedings, Folder: Joint Convention (Dists 1, 7, 9)—1903, Indiana University of Pennsylvania, Archives and Special Collections.

While parts of the decision probably will not suit: "Editor Mine Workers' Journal," *Wilkes-Barre Semi-Weekly Record*, March 24, 1903.

The arbitration commission concludes that the Coal and Iron Police should be disbanded: Anthracite Coal Strike Commission, "Report to the President on the of Anthracite Coal Strike," 83.

We must *have peace and order*: Anthracite Coal Strike Commission, "Report to the President on the Anthracite Coal Strike," 84.

Conclusion: A Wrecking Crew

patrolled the streets of Mauch Chunk with loaded rifles: Robert V. Bruce, 1877, Year of Violence (Chicago: Ivan R. Dee Publishers, 1989), 67.

inauguration of a new order of things: "Our County Politics," *Scranton Tribune*, July 30, 1874.

***We could have routed* them all:** "Wednesday's Sad Event," *Scranton Republican*, August 8, 1877.

***Citizen soldiers should not be called on*:** "Misuse of the National Guard," Philadelphia *Times*, August 4, 1892.

our inefficient method of enforcing the law: "State Constabulary," *Wilkes-Barre Semi-Weekly Record*, October 22, 1897.

The sheriff, and even the deputies: "Drift in Politics," Scranton Times, December 11, 1897.

The road to the institution of police was paved in the *mad days of riot*: "Military and Masonic Pageant," *Scranton Republican*, November 21, 1877.

Like the *Easton Greys* in 1877: "Regulars at Reading," *Harrisburg Telegraph*, July 25, 1877.

to keep the labor-friendly newspapers from stirring *up the mob elements*: "Vigilantes after the Newspapers," *Harrisburg Telegraph*, July 25, 1877.

***Law and Order Brigade*:** "Law's Triumph," Philadelphia *Times*, July 28, 1877.

and then built it atop their mine: Joseph J. Holmes, "The Decline of the Pennsylvania Militia: 1815–1870," *The Western Pennsylvania Historical Magazine* 57, no. 2 (April 1974): 213.

They built armories for the vigilantes: John K. Mahon, *History of the Militia and the National Guard* (New York: Macmillan, 1983), 113; Holmes, "The Decline of The Pennsylvania Militia," 210.

The Lackawanna Iron and Coal Co. donated land: Holmes, "The Decline of The Pennsylvania Militia," 199.

The Reading Railroad built spurs to militia encampments: Holmes, "The Decline of The Pennsylvania Militia," 198.

***private police force of industry*:** Mahon, *History of the Militia and the National Guard*, 116; Holmes, "The Decline of The Pennsylvania Militia," 200, 283; Matthew Margis, "America's Progressive Army: How the National Guard Grew out of Progressive Era Reforms" (PhD diss., Iowa State University, 2016), 10.

always left them in the lurch after a strike: Herbert D. Croly, *The Promise of American Life* (New York: Macmillan, 1912), 344; "A State Constabulary," *Wilkes-Barre Times Leader*, June 19, 1894.

always came with *frightful consequences*: "Drift in Politics."

***hideous class hatreds* and lasting *enmity*:** "State Constabulary," *Wilkes-Barre Semi-Weekly Record*, October 22, 1897; "Drift in Politics"; Bruce, *1877, Year of Violence*, 18; Gary Jones, "American Cossacks: The Pennsylvania Department of State Police and Labor, 1890–1917" (PhD diss., Lehigh University, 1997), 6; "A State Constabulary," *Wilkes-Barre Times Leader*, June 19, 1894.

the militias and Pinkertons and sheriff's posses: "A State Constabulary," *Wilkes-Barre Times Leader*, June 19, 1894.

***creation of a state constabulary*:** "Along the lines of the highly trained and disciplined constabulary of Pennsylvania to aid the local police or constabulary in repressing disorder." Margis, "America's Progressive Army," 39 and 274; "Says Unions Hurt Militia," *New York Times*, November 15, 1910.

protect people outside of the cities against violent crimes: "A State Constabulary," *Altoona Tribune*, January 10, 1901.

***run down criminals wherever they may flee*:** "A State Constabulary"; "Drift in Politics"; "A Needed Force," Sacramento *Record-Union*, February 25, 1889.

vested interests and free from *party politics*: "Misuse of the National Guard," Philadelphia *Times*, August 4, 1892; "A Needed Force," *Sacramento Record-Union*, February 25, 1889; "Rich Plums for Platt," Baltimore *Sun*, November 12, 1900.

even the strikers, would benefit: "Drift in Politics."

could be tutored in the ***just rights of labor, as well as property*****:** "Drift in Politics."

the ***powder and shot*** **of the militia:** "A State Constabulary," Wilkes-Barre *Times*, June 19, 1894.

a state ***constabulary could be called*****:** "A State Constabulary and the Forests," *Philadelphia Inquirer*, August 6, 1892.

trained for both preventive and repressive service**:** "Misuse of the National Guard," Philadelphia *Times*, August 4, 1892.

the result will be ***bruised heads*****:** "A State Constabulary," Wilkes-Barre *Times*, June 19, 1894.

Had there been a small force of regularly organized State constabulary: "State Constabulary," *Wilkes-Barre Semi-Weekly Record*, October 22, 1897.

their pleas were always left unheeded: Jones, "American Cossacks," 6.

New Hampshire voters overwhelmingly rejected a state constabulary: "Heavy Majority Against the State Constabulary Act," *Philadelphia Inquirer*, November 11, 1869.

California tried and failed in 1880: "The State Constabulary Bill," Sacramento *Record-Union*, April 14, 1880.

newspapers called him a ***Czar*****:** "St. John's Constabulary," *Wichita Daily Times*, June 26, 1882.

New York State tried and failed to pass a state constabulary law: "State Constabulary Bill: Legislature Awaiting the Measure Now in Preparation," *New York Times*, April 11, 1899; "State Police," *Carbondale News*, November 22, 1900; "State Police," Brooklyn *Standard Union*, March 22, 1899. Some states had what they called a state constabulary. Maine and Massachusetts created a statewide force in the 1860s, Rhode Island in 1874, and Michigan in 1880, but all these were limited to the enforcement of liquor laws only: see "To Enforce Liquor Laws," *Chicago Tribune*, May 7, 1887; "First Words," *Boston Evening Transcript*, May 16, 1867; "Review of the Week," *New England Farmer*, June 6, 1874.

shoot down striking workmen in the name of the law**:** "Labor vs. Militia," *Rocky Mountain News*, December 2, 1897, as quoted in Margis, "America's Progressive Army," 50.

promised ***to replace the Coal and Iron Police*****:** Gerda Ray, "From Cossack to Trooper: Manliness, Police Reform, and the State." *Journal of Social History* 28, no. 3 (1995): 566; see Samuel W. Pennypacker, *Autobiography of a Pennsylvanian* (Philadelphia: Winston & Co., 1918); Katherine Mayo, *Justice to All: The Story of the Pennsylvania State Police* (New York:

G. P. Putnam's Sons, 1917).

independent of our orders: Jones, "American Cossacks," 37.

the bill became law: Created by P.L. 361 May 2, 1905.

the bill describes it as a rural constabulary: "More Laws and Salaries," *Gettysburg Compiler*, May 31, 1905, p. 3.

admirable model: "Pennsylvania's State Constabulary," *The Nation*, July 20, 1905, pp. 49–50.

They fought strikers at Homestead in 1892: Report of the Adjutant General of Pennsylvania for the Year Ended December 31, 1906 (Harrisburg: State Printer, 1908), 10, 17.

He steamed to Dublin in September 1905: Letter from John C. Groome to Gov. Pennypacker, August 22, 1905, MG-171-4: Pennypacker Papers, Box 50: Executive Correspondence, Folder: Executive Correspondence, 1904–06, Penn State Police, Groome, John C. (Supt.), Pennsylvania State Archives, Harrisburg, PA. "Groome Coming Home," *Philadelphia Inquirer*, September 27, 1905. On the role of the constabulary in the Irish Land War, see Brian O'Neill, *The War for the Land in Ireland* (New York: International Publishers, 1933). On the origins, tactics, and campaigns of the RIC, see Vicky Collins, *Policing Twentieth Century Ireland: A History of An Garda Síochána* (New York: Routledge, 2014).

Pennsylvania State Police *will be in every sense of the word military police*: "New State Police Force," *Allentown Leader*, September 8, 1902.

men accustomed to war and detectives' work: "The State's Constabulary," *Fulton County News*, September 6, 1905.

He would outfit each trooper with: Jones, "American Cossacks," 54; Annual Report of 1908, January 1 1908, Box 4, Folder 3: Records of the Pennsylvania State Police, RG-030: Records of the State Police, Series 30.2; Game Commission, 1918–1945; Governor's File, 1905–1915, Pennsylvania State Archives, Harrisburg.

He mounted his troopers on horses: Annual Report of 1905, December 31, 1906, RG-030: Records of the Pennsylvania State Police Series, Series 30.2; Game Commission, 1918–1945; Governor's File, 1905–1915, Box 4, Folder 3: Records of the PA State Police, Pennsylvania State Archives, Harrisburg, PA; Jones, "American Cossacks," 13.

The farmers are pretty tame: "Captain Groome Talks of Constabulary," *Philadelphia Inquirer*, September 30, 1905.

Two troops occupied the western bituminous fields: Testimony of Maurer, to the Commission on Industrial Relations, in "Final Report and Testimony,"

Vol. XI (Washington: Gov't Printing Office, 1912), p. 10,976; Jones, "American Cossacks," 53, 57.

***Pennypacker's Cossacks,* his *Black Hussars*:** Holmes, "The Decline of The Pennsylvania Militia," 282.

predicted *a brutal constabulary*: Mother Jones, *The Autobiography of Mother Jones*. Edited by Mary Field Parton, introduction by Clarence Darrow. Charles H. Kerr Publishing Company, 1925, 60.

not like anyone can *tell a so-called striker*: Testimony of John C. Groome, Superintendent, Pennsylvania State Police, to the Commission on Industrial Relations, in "Final Report and Testimony," Vol. XI (Washington: Gov't Printing Office, 1912), p. 10969.

***outnumbered by the lawless element*:** Annual Report of 1905, December 31, 1906, RG-030: Records of the Pennsylvania State Police Series; Series 30.2; Game Commission, 1918–1945; Governor's File, 1905–1915, Box 4, Folder 3: Records of the Pennsylvania State Police, Pennsylvania State Archives, Harrisburg, PA.

***unsettled condition of affairs in the Anthracite Region*:** Special Order No. 13, 26 April 1906, MG-171-4: Pennypacker Papers, Box 50: Executive Correspondence, Folder: Executive Correspondence, 1904–06, Penn State Police, Groome, John C. (Supt.), Pennsylvania State Archives, Harrisburg, PA; *Wilkes-Barre Semi-Weekly Record*, April 10 1906, "Pipe Line Dynamited" and "Connell will Accept."

***foreign colony near the Fernwood colliery*:** Special Order No. 13, April 26 1906, MG-171-4: Pennypacker Papers, Box 50: Executive Correspondence, Folder: Executive Correspondence, 1904–06, Penn State Police, Groome, John C. (Supt.), Pennsylvania State Archives, Harrisburg, PA; *Wilkes-Barre Semi-Weekly Record*, April 10 1906, "Pipe Line Dynamited" and "Connell will Accept."

they *shackled* striking miners *in irons*: "Warrant Was Issued for Lehigh Valley Official Perjury Is Charge Named," *Wilkes-Barre News*, April 14, 1906.

we'd prefer to go *in and club the hell out of them*: Letter from J. B. Cheyney, *Wilkes-Barre Times Leader*, April 5, 1906, MG-171-4: Governor Pennypacker Papers, Box 50: Executive Correspondence, Folder: Executive Correspondence, 1904–06, Penn State Police, Groome, John C. (Supt.), Pennsylvania State Archives, Harrisburg, PA.

people he'd *return and burn the place to the ground*: Letter from J. B. Cheyney, *Wilkes-Barre Times Leader*, April 10, 1906, MG-171-4: Governor Pennypacker Papers, Box 50: Executive Correspondence, Folder: Executive Correspondence, 1904–06, Penna State Police, Groome, John C. (Supt.), Pennsylvania State Archives, Harrisburg, PA.

These are military men: "Status of the State Police," *Wilkes-Barre News*, April 7, 1906.

guarding the constables: Annual Report of 1908, January 1, 1908, Box 4, Folder 3: Records of the Pennsylvania State Police, RG-030: Records of the State Police, Series 30.2; Game Commission, 1918–1945; Governor's File, 1905–1915, Pennsylvania State Archives, Harrisburg; *Philadelphia Inquirer*, May 21, 1908, "Chester Police to Help Operate Trolley Cars."

Undercover state cops infiltrated the strikers: Testimony of James H. Maurer, President, Pennsylvania State Federation of Labor, Commission on Industrial Relations, in "Final Report and Testimony," Vol. XI (Washington: Government Printing Office, 1912), p. 10,933; "Hazleton Trolley Strike," *Mauch Chunk Daily Times*, April 10, 1914.

conditions were *worse than in 1902*: Comment of Adam Ryscavage, President, UMW District 1, Transcript of Proceedings of the Conference Between Representatives of the Anthracite Coal Operators and Representatives of the Anthracite Mine Workers, Philadelphia, PA, March 11 and 12 and April 7 and 9, 1908, Collection MG 109, Series 3: Office Records, Subseries B, Box 8: Anthracite Wage Agreements, Archives and Special Collections, Indiana University of Pennsylvania, Indiana, PA.

the Chamber of Commerce *created a Committee for State Police*: Ray, "From Cossack to Trooper," 566–67.

***Life in the outlying and sparsely settled districts*:** Lewis Rutherford Morris, Chairman Committee for a New York State Police, "State Police Protection in Country Districts Essential to Development" RG-030: Records of the Pennsylvania State Police Series; 30.13: Historical File, Box 2, Folder 7, Pennsylvania State Archive, Harrisburg, PA.

They brought in Groome to speak: Ray, "From Cossack to Trooper," 569.

who would later defend colonialism in her 1927 book *Mother India*: Katherine Mayo, *Mother India* (New York: Praeger, 1927).

***onslaught of rural crime* by violent immigrants and blacks:** Ray, "From Cossack to Trooper," 569.

She testified before state commissions: Ray, "From Cossack to Trooper," 568.

The campaign culminated in her 1917 book *Justice to All*: Katherine Mayo, *Justice to All: The Story of the Pennsylvania State Police* (New York: G. P. Putnam's Sons, 1917).

rioting mobs of foreigners: Mayo, *Justice to All*, xv, 141.

***hordes of savage Huns* and *mercurial* Italians and Poles:** Mayo, *Justice to All*, 79.

Whenever the miners elected to go out on strike: Mayo, *Justice to All*, 2.

the lawless capitalists who used the law-defying Coal and Iron Police: Mayo, *Justice to All*, ix–x.

New York created a state constabulary in 1917: Ray, "From Cossack to Trooper," 565.

the drifting smoke and soot of police had settled everywhere: Paul Musgrave, "Bringing the State Police In: The Diffusion of US Statewide Policing Agencies, 1905–1941," *Studies in American Political Development* 34, no. 1 (2020): 3–23.

How did the Pennsylvania State Police protect: Various reports of Agent #607. RG-030: Records of the Pennsylvania State Police, Series 30: Strike Reports, Box 1: Strike Reports, 1922–1950, Folder: Bureau of Crime, Strike Reports, Western PA.

They forged union cards: Reports of Agent #607, May 11, 1922, RG-030: Records of the Pennsylvania State Police, Series 30: Strike Reports, Box 1: Strike Reports, 1922–1950, Folder: Bureau of Crime, Strike Reports, Western PA; Coal, April 26–September 5, 1922, Pennsylvania State Archives, Harrisburg, PA.

wrote reports about *how much liquor*: Reports of Agent #607, April 30, 1922, RG-030: Records of the Pennsylvania State Police, Series 30: Strike Reports, Box 1: Strike Reports, 1922–1950, Folder: Bureau of Crime, Strike Reports, Western PA; Coal, April 26–September 5, 1922, Pennsylvania State Archives, Harrisburg, PA.

rumors of *dynamite buried in the hills*: Reports of Agent #607, May 11, 1922, RG-030: Records of the Pennsylvania State Police, Series 30: Strike Reports, Box 1: Strike Reports, 1922–1950, Folder: Bureau of Crime, Strike Reports, Western PA; Coal, April 26–September 5, 1922, Pennsylvania State Archives, Harrisburg, PA.

strikers' secret plots to *give battle to the State Police*: Reports of Agent #607, April 29, 1922, RG-030: Records of the Pennsylvania State Police, Series 30: Strike Reports, Box 1: Strike Reports, 1922–1950, Folder: Bureau of Crime, Strike Reports, Western PA; Coal, April 26–September 5, 1922, Pennsylvania State Archives, Harrisburg, PA.

every *man is armed* whether they were or not: Reports of Agent #607, April 29, 1922, RG-030: Records of the Pennsylvania State Police, Series 30: Strike Reports, Box 1: Strike Reports, 1922–1950, Folder: Bureau of Crime, Strike Reports, Western PA; Coal, April 26–September 5, 1922, Pennsylvania State Archives, Harrisburg, PA.

***foreigners are becoming restless*:** Reports of Agent #607, May 4, 1922 & May

5, 1922, RG-030: Records of the Pennsylvania State Police, Series 30: Strike Reports, Box 1: Strike Reports, 1922–1950, Folder: Bureau of Crime, Strike Reports, Western PA; Coal, April 26–September 5, 1922, Pennsylvania State Archives, Harrisburg, PA.

more private deputies must be brought on: Report of Agent #607, 7 May 1922, RG-030: Records of the Pennsylvania State Police, Series 30: Strike Reports, Box 1: Strike Reports, 1922–1950, Folder: Bureau of Crime, Strike Reports, Western PA; Coal, April 26–September 5, 1922, Pennsylvania State Archives, Harrisburg, PA.

The *loafers* and *young rowdies*: Reports of Agent #607, April 30, 1922, RG-030: Records of the Pennsylvania State Police, Series 30: Strike Reports, Box 1: Strike Reports, 1922–1950, Folder: Bureau of Crime, Strike Reports, Western PA; Coal, April 26–September 5, 1922, Pennsylvania State Archives, Harrisburg, PA.

***What is needed in this vicinity*:** Reports of Agent #607, April 26, 1922, RG-030: Records of the Pennsylvania State Police, Series 30: Strike Reports, Box 1: Strike Reports, 1922–1950, Folder: Bureau of Crime, Strike Reports, Western PA; Coal, April 26–September 5, 1922, Pennsylvania State Archives, Harrisburg, PA.

trucks mounted with large-caliber machine guns: Intelligence Bulletin No. 17, August 14, 1922, 104th Cavalry Headquarters, Camp Crooks, Cokeburg, RG-030: Records of the Pennsylvania State Police, Series 30: Strike Reports, Box 1: Strike Reports, 1922–1950, Folder: Bureau of Crime, Strike Reports, Western PA; Coal, April 26–September 5, 1922, Pennsylvania State Archives, Harrisburg, PA.

***commanding a field of fire*:** Intelligence Bulletin No. 3, July 29, 1922, Pennsylvania National Guard, Headquarters 104th Cavalry, Camp Crooks, Cokeburg, RG-030: Records of the Pennsylvania State Police, Series 30: Strike Reports, Box 1: Strike Reports, 1922–1950, Folder: Bureau of Crime, Strike Reports, Western PA; Coal, April 26–September 5, 1922, Pennsylvania State Archives, Harrisburg, PA.

terrifying the strikers and driving them away: Intelligence Bulletin No. 16, August 13, 1922, 104th Cavalry Headquarters, Camp Crooks, Cokeburg, RG-030: Records of the Pennsylvania State Police, Series 30: Strike Reports, Box 1: Strike Reports, 1922–1950, Folder: Bureau of Crime, Strike Reports, Western PA; Coal, April 26–September 5, 1922, Pennsylvania State Archives, Harrisburg, PA.

arrested and held strike leaders without bail: Intelligence Bulletin No. 10, August 5, 1922, Pennsylvania National Guard, Headquarters 104th Cavalry, Camp Crooks, Cokeburg, RG-030: Records of the Pennsylvania State

Police, Series 30: Strike Reports, Box 1: Strike Reports, 1922–1950, Folder: Bureau of Crime, Strike Reports, Western PA; Coal, April 26–September 5, 1922, Pennsylvania State Archives, Harrisburg, PA.

They embedded special agents: See RG-030: Records of the Pennsylvania State Police, Series 30: Strike Reports, Box 1: Strike Reports, 1922–1950, Pennsylvania State Archives, Harrisburg, PA.

***begging the farmers for food*:** Intelligence Bulletin No. 7, August 1922, Pennsylvania National Guard, Headquarters 104th Cavalry, Camp Crooks, Cokeburg, RG-030: Records of the Pennsylvania State Police, Series 30: Strike Reports, Box 1: Strike Reports, 1922–1950, Folder: Bureau of Crime, Strike Reports, Western PA; Coal, April 26–September 5, 1922, Pennsylvania State Archives, Harrisburg, PA.

epidemic of ruptured backs and torn Achilles that followed: Minutes of Special Convention of Territory 6, District 2, held at Indiana, PA, November 7, 1920, Collection 52, Series I: United Mine Workers of America, Box 1: Early Records, Folder 16: Reports and minutes, 1920–21, Archives and Special Collections, Indiana University of Pennsylvania, Indiana, PA.

***weak-kneed workers* joined up with the foremen:** Minutes of Council of Action Convention, Froshinn Theater, Altoona, PA, February 22, 1921, Collection 52, Series I: United Mine Workers of America, Folder 16: Reports and minutes, 1920–21, Archives and Special Collections, Indiana University of Pennsylvania, Indiana, PA.

employers have *declared war upon the working class of this country*: Minutes of Council of Action Convention, Froshinn Theater, Altoona, PA, February 22, 1921, Collection 52, Series I: United Mine Workers of America, Folder 16: Reports and minutes, 1920–21, Archives and Special Collections, Indiana University of Pennsylvania, Indiana, PA.

militant miners, they complained, *swarmed into the coalfields*: United Mine Workers of America, "Attempt by Communists to Seize the American Labor Movement," National Capital Press, Washington, DC, 1923, pp. 8, 14, 20.

purged all those who challenged Lewis: United Mine Workers of America, "Attempt by Communists to Seize the American Labor Movement," National Capital Press, Washington, DC, 1923, p. 3.

If you fellows in Pennsylvania had kicked up the same: Philip S. Foner, *History of the Labor Movement in the United States: The T.U.E.L. to the End of the Gompers Era*, vol. 9, (New York, International Publishers, 1991), 220; Anonymous Letter, June 15, 1923, Collection 52: Early Records, United Mine Workers of American, District 2, Series I: United Mine Workers of America, Box 2, Series I, Folder 7 Various items on Coal Mining, n.d.,

Archives and Special Collections, Indiana University of Pennsylvania, Indiana, PA.

***ran wild over western Pennsylvania*:** "Civil Union Opens Probe Into Strike," *Wilkes-Barre Times Leader*, May 21, 1935; Seth Low, president of the National Civic Federation, surprised the miners' union when he supported the creation of the New York State Police. See Ray, "From Cossack to Trooper," 567.

evicted them by tearing the roofs off: Testimony of Lowell F. Limpus, Reporter, *New York Daily News,* "Conditions in the Coalfields of Pennsylvania, West Virginia, and Ohio," Hearings Before the Committee on Interstate Commerce, United States Senate, Vol. 1, Gov. Printing Office, Washington, DC, 1928, pp. 940–50.

The union preached patience: Testimony of Lowell F. Limpus, Reporter, *New York Daily News,* "Conditions in the Coalfields of Pennsylvania, West Virginia, and Ohio," Hearings Before the Committee on Interstate Commerce, United States Senate, Vol. 1, Gov. Printing Office, Washington, DC, 1928, p. 942.

***the treatment of police was good*:** "Civil Union Opens Probe Into Strike," *Wilkes-Barre Times Leader*, May 21, 1935; Walter T. Howard, "The National Miners Union: Communists and Miners in the Pennsylvania Anthracite, 1928–1931," *The Pennsylvania Magazine of History and Biography* 125, no. 1 and 2 (2001): 93–94; "Terror in Pennsylvania," *New Republic*, August 21, 1935.

torturing them until they signed blank cards on which the police later typed the words the treatment of police was good: "Civil Union Opens Probe Into Strike," *Wilkes-Barre Times Leader*, May 21, 1935.

***They're all in the same nest*:** "Civil Union Opens Probe Into Strike."

***Some men had their heads busted*:** "Terror in Pennsylvania," *New Republic*, August 21, 1935, p. 35.

INDEX

Adams, Lynn G., 193
agencies, detective, 37, 53, 58, 60, 103, 108, 113. *See also* police
agents, labor, 28, 99, 101, 145
Alabama, 8
Allen, Necho, 44, 45
American Federation of Labor, 150
Ancient Order of the Hibernians. *See* Molly Maguires
Anthracite Coal Operators Association, 75
Anthracite Coal Strike Commission, 161–180; appointment of, 161, 162; decision of, 178, 179; fact-finding tour of, 163
Archibald Benevolent Association, 51
arks, 22, 46, 47; building of, 46; use for, 47. *See also* rafts
Ashland, 134, 141
assimilation, 67, 75, 130
Auchincloss, 107
Audenried, 163
Baer, George, 39, 81, 147, 149
Baker, Mike, 165
Baltimore, 53,
Bates, John, 50
Battle of a Thousand Slain, 45, 46. *See also* St. Clair's Defeat; Battle of the Wabash River
Battle of the Wabash River, 45, 46. *See also* St. Clair's Defeat; Battle of a Thousand Slain
Beaver Meadow, 58, 121–123, 127
Beddall, Joseph, 133, 134, 140
Beddall, Rowland, 133, 140
Beddall, Thomas, 131–134
Benevolent Society of Carbon County, 51, 186
black damp, 15, 30, 34
blacklegs, 56, 107; ballad of the, 57
blacklist, x, 11, 25–28, 36, 40, 63, 69, 72, 87, 93, 103, 124, 127, 131, 150–153, 168
Black Tuesday, 60. *See also*, Molly Maguires; Day of the Rope

Blairsville, 99
boardinghouse, 1–3, 26, 75, 76, 144; Blussick's, 1–3
bobtail check, 19, 29. *See also* miners, anthracite: wages of
Borcoski, John, 2, 3; arrest of, 3, 4; children of, 6; death of, 5; funeral of, 6; torture of, 2–5
Borcoski, Sofia, 5; burial of husband by, 6; search for husband by, 5, 6; settlement for husband's death, 6
bosses: aggressive nature of, 37; barking orders of the, 32, 37; blacklisting of the, x, 11, 25–28, 36, 40, 63, 69, 72, 87, 93, 103, 124, 127, 131, 150–153, 168 72; burning hatred for, 60, 103, 104; docking by the, 21, 22, 32, 36, 39, 50–52, 150; incompetence of, 62; murderous, 34, 35, 41, 55; thugs recruited by, 29; violence of, 23, 32–36 37, 40-42, 64, 165, 166, 173, 184. *See also* souls of capital, rotten
boycott, 103, 117, 125
Boyle, James, 60
breaker boy, x, 25, 30, 37, 62, 69, 73, 80, 99, 103–105, 179, 134, 156, 165, 166
breaker, 30, 37, 48, 62, 103, 112, 154, 163–166
Broad Mountain, 44
Brotherhood of Railroad Fireman, the, 108
Brown, John, 59
Buckongahelas, 45
Burns, Kate, 40
Business Men's Association, 145

California, 184
Campbell, Alexander, 60
canals: Chesapeake and Tidewater, 48; coal shipped by, 22, 48; competition between railroads and, 48, 50; Delaware and Hudson, 48; Delaware Division, 48; Morris, 48; Pennsylvania, 48; Schuylkill Navigation, 48
Carbon County, 110
Carnegie, Andrew, 28
Carroll, James, 60
Caruso, Patsy, 3
Carboniferous Period, 20, 44
Catawissa Valley, 138
cavalry 8, 110, 131, 134, 137, 138, 144, 146, 185, 186, 190
Central Railroad of New Jersey, 107
Centralia, 140
Cherokee, 45
Cheslak, Mike, 65
Chester, 187
Chicago, 26, 97 113
Chippie, Andrew, 40, 166
Cincinnati, 26, 45
Citizen Corps, 182
Citizen's Alliance, 130, 140–143
Civil War, 50, 52, 90, 91, 92, 136
Clark, E.E., 161
coal, anthracite: adoption of,

8, 9, 22, 23, 46–51; brokers and dealers of, 22, 62, 74, 99, 145; burning of, 9, 23, 74; face of, 15, 16, 173; geography of, 8–11, 15; geological formation of, 44; industrial development by, 9–11, 23, 50; influence on mammoth vein of, 129; military interest in, 9, 50; pillars of, 35; price of, 54, 55, 99, 145; stored energy of, 16, 20; total mined of, 37, 50, 51; transportation of, 22, 46–49; uniqueness of, 23, 32, 50, 51; veins of, 15, 16, 21, 23, 34, 52, 129, 173
coal, bituminous, 80, 88, 98, 145
coalcrackers, ix
Coal Miners' and Laborers' National Progressive Union, 63
Coleman Guards, 136
Coleraine, 123
Coll, Henry, 30, 31, 32, 151, 155, 156–159; eviction of, 155–159; injury history of, 155
Coll, Mary, 155–159; death of, 159
collieries: attacks on, 56, 105, 106, 107, 141, 143, 144; description of 23, 24, 101, 135, 154; role of police at, 57, 100, 108, 109, 110, 111, 116, 144, 146, 153
companies, coal. *See* operators, coal
Connecticut, 8, 26, 189
conquest: cowardice and, 45; property and, 44, 135, 136
Coverdale, 192
Coxe Bros. & Co., 58, 64, 65, 108–110, 115, 116, 146, 155
Cranberry colliery, 152, 177
Cresco, 177
culm pickers, 35–37, 58, 62, 76
culm banks, 27, 35, 56, 61, 62, 75, 100, 101, 129, 132, 138; exploding of, 61, 106, 107
Cushma, Mike, 158; eviction of, 158

Damensko, John, 65
Davis, David, 19
Day of the Rope, 60. *See also* Molly Maguires; Black Tuesday
Death, Angel of, 33. *See also* inspector, mine
Delaware, 189
Demko, John, 171
Derr, Jerry, 117
Derringer, 117
Draper colliery, 144
Drinkwater, John, 142
Darrow, Clarence, 162–180
Debs, Eugene V., 162
Delaware, Lackawanna & Western Railroad, 48
Delaware River, 43
Delaware, Susquehanna & Schuylkill Railroad, 110,
Dettery, William, 40, 41, 117, 118, 125, 126
Dolan, Thomas, 142
Donahue, John, 60
Douglass, Frederick, 59

Doyle, Michael, 60
Drifton colliery, 58, 110–112, 115–120, 137, 146, 163
Dublin, 185
Duffy, Thomas, 60, 76, 112, 152
Dunleavy, Paul, 151, 156, 158; eviction of, 156, 157
Duryea, 26, 99

East Millsboro, 190
Easton, 48
Easton Greys, 182
Eckert, Isaac, 109, 116, 118
enslavement, 59. *See also* miners, anthracite: wages of
effigy, 1, 2, 12, 104, 105, 117, 122
Egushaway, 45
Evans, Billy, 113–128, methods of, 113, 114, 122–126
Evans, Daniel, 170

Fahy, John, 97
Fernwood colliery, 186
Filler, Gottlieb, 153
firedamp, 20
First Troop Philadelphia City Cavalry, 185
Flynn, Bartholomew, 113, 118, 119
Forestville Improvement Society, 51
Frackville, 141
Franklin colliery, 187
Fredericksburg, Battle of, 91
Freeland, 58, 73, 74, 115, 119, 120, 151
funiculars (railroad), 47

Gallagher, James (half-dead), 29–36, 39, 82, 152, 153, 157; eviction of, 157
Gelgot, William, 115, 116
Georgia, 8, 136
Gilberton, 129, 144
Gimshock, John, 152
Gobin, John, P.S., 106, 134–147
Gompers, Samuel, 13, 150
Gordon, John, 122–124
Governor's Troop of the Pennsylvania Cavalry, 110
Gowen Compromise, 54–56
Gowen, Franklin, 54–60
Gray, George, 161–162, 170, 176
Groome, John C., 185–193

Hannik, Andrew, 29, 33, 39, 152, 158; eviction of, 158
Harrisburg, 136, 137, 182
Hartlein, George, 88, 89
Harvilla, John, 121–123
Haymarket Affair, the, 113
Hazleton, 26, 27, 42, 45, 57, 68, 72–100, 106, 111–113, 129, 137, 145, 146, 156–158, 163, 177, 185
Helferty, Charlie, 40, 42, 151, 157; eviction of, 157
Henderson, 190
Hermany, Will, 125, 126
Higgins, John, 2, 3
Hollenback Mine, 49, 105
Homestead, 181, 185
Honeybrook colliery, 63
houses, company, 40, 75, 99
houses, alms and poor, 41, 99, 167–169

Howat, Alexander, 191, 192
Hudock, John, 119, 125, 126
Huns, 26, 129, 130, 189. *See also* miners, coal: slurs used against

Illinois, 8, 36, 38 162,
immigration: descriptions of 24–29
immigrants: arrival of, 24–26; depictions of, 75, 76, 129–131, 171, 172, 188, 190; homelands of 24, 25, 75; institutions built by, 27; living conditions for, 75, 76, 129–132, 173; organizing by, 63, 64, 65, 104; policing of, 186, 187; radicalism of, 64; reasons for migrating by, 24, 25; role in union, 104
Indiana, 8
inspectors, mining, 20, 33, 34; hatred of, 26, 27
Iowa, 8, 81

Jacquott, Charles, 152, 157; eviction of, 157
James, John, 114, 119, 120
Jeddo, 29, 39, 42, 98, 137, 151–159, 163, 175
John, Ezekiel, 142
Jones, Gomer, 63
Jones, Mother, 150, 186, 192

Kahley, Frank, 126
Kamjuck, Anthony, 152
Kansas, 184
Keenan, Charles, 152, 158; eviction of, 158
Kelly, Edward, 60
Kentucky, 8
Knights of Labor, 36, 63
Korkosky, Stiney, 134
Krezo, George, 65
Kulich, John, 65

Lackawanna Iron and Coal Company, 182
Lanigan's colliery, 133
Lansford, 143, 144
Lattimer, 64, 65,
Lattimer Massacre, 63–65, 96, 97, 137, 174–176, 183
Laurel Run Improvement Company, 55
Law and Order Brigade, 182
law: martial, 134; police and, 114; private property and, 44; violence and, 60, 97, 98, 181
Lehigh and Wilkes-Barre Coal Company, 107, 154
Lehigh Coal and Navigation Company, 174, 179
Lehigh Coal Company, 46, 154
Lehigh River, 43, 44, 46, 47
Lehigh Valley, 161, 177
Lehigh Valley Coal Company, 63, 137
Lehigh Valley Railroad, 48, 110
Lewis, John L., 191
Lenni Lenape, 43, 45
Lewis, Shadrach, 170
Lincoln, Abraham, 59,
Little Schuylkill River, 44, 47

Luzerne County, 41, 57, 58, 109, 110, 154, 186
Lyster, Walter: murder of Borcoski by, 4,5; prosecution for murder of Borcoski by, 6; torture of Borcoski by, 4, 5

Mahanoy City, 131, 137, 140, 145, 146, 179
Maine, 8
Maloney, Thomas, 193
Maltby colliery, 144
Markle, G.B. & Co., 40, 151–155, 166, 179
Markle, John, 80, 151–157, 161, 166, 179
Martin, James, 64, 65, 105, 175
Marx, Karl, 59
Massachusetts, 26
Mauch Chunk, 60, 137, 181
Maxilon, Fandishaf, 65
Mayo, Katherine, 188, 189, defense of colonialism by, 188
McAdoo, 63, 74, 79, 80
McCann, Charlie, 107
McCarthy, D.J., 153, 154, 175
McDonigle, Neal, 20
McEmoyle, Hugh, 142–144
McGehan, Hugh, 60
McKelvey, Daniel, 111–113
McParland, James, 60
Mellon, Andrew, 28
Mellon family, 6
Midlick, Mike, 40
migration, 24–26, 73, 74; return, 73, 99; use of steamships for, 25, 26, 67, 99
militia, 56, 136, 140, 144, 181–187. *See also* Pennsylvania National Guard
mines, bootleg, 58
Miners' Benevolent Society of Locust Gap, 51
Miners' Journal, The, 66
Miners and Laborers' Amalgamated Association, 63
miners, anthracite: blacklisting of, 11 25, 28, 87, 93, 94, 151–153; children of, 12, 29, 35–37, 58, 99, 165, 166, 171; contract, 18, 26, 28, 52, 163, 166, 171; cost of tools borne by, 18, 19; cribbing by, 21; descriptions of, 23–29; divisions among, 28, 51, 52; docking of, 21, 22, 32, 36, 39, 50–52, 150; ethnicity of 11, 25, 26; eviction of, 28, 99, 131, 149–159, 162, 185; illnesses of, 24, 167–170; injuries to, 32, 40–42, 71, 167–170, 191; living conditions of, 75, 76, 168–173, 191; lungs of, 5, 17, 24, 168, 169; patience required of, 16–19; recruitment of, 25–27; skills of, 16–23, 34; slurs used against, 26, 129–131, 189; solidarity of, 11, 12, 28, 69, 77, 78, 104, 131; strike tactics of, 12, 103–106, 111, 112, 141; use of violence in strikes by, 12, 29, 103;

wages of, 21, 23, 29, 30, 40, 49, 52–56, 59, 69, 75, 99, 163–167, 170–174, 178, 183, 191; wealth created by, 28, 36, 37, 165; working conditions of, 15–24, 165–170, 191
Minersville, 146
mining: brattices used in, 16, 17, 20; causes of accidents in, 16–22, 29–35, 40–42, 165–175; coal cars used in, 20–23, 39–41, 69, 70, 173, 191; dangers of, 11, 17–20, 30–32, 49, 71, 93, 94, 163–180; differences in methods in, 16–22, 52; methods in, 15–20, 29, 30, 165–170; risks of listening to bosses in, 18, 32, 41; role of docking bosses in, 21, 22; types of openings for, 15; use of explosives in, 16, 18, 19, 20, 78, 166
Minnesota, 8
Mishikinaakwa, 45
Mitchell, John, 13, 36, 37, 66–71, 73–100, 140, 146–150, 162–163, 179; commission testimony of, 163, 164
Mocanaqua, 187
Molly Maguires, 52, 59–61, 95, 129, 130, 137, 138, 181
Morgan, J.P., 28, 48, 147, 161
Morris, Milner T., 65
Mt. Carmel, 146
Mt. Gretna, 136
Mulraney, Dan, 115, 118, 119–121
Munley, Thomas, 60
Musmanno, Michael: campaign to abolish private police by, 7, 10; lawsuit against Mellon family by, 6; legal defense of Sofia Borcoski by, 7; politics of, 1, 10; research into private policing by, 7
Mutual Beneficial Association, 191

Nanticoke, 27, 116
Nation, The, 185
National Civic Federation, 38, 66, 70, 71, 81, 95, 96
National Trade Assembly 135, 63
Nesquehoning, 141, 143, 145
New Hampshire, 184
New Jersey, 189
New Philadelphia, 146
New York, 25, 26, 28, 48, 68, 70, 74, 81, 85, 86, 89, 97–100, 147, 184, 188, 189
Nichols, T.D., 68, 88
Nohie, John, 152
North Carolina, 8
North Dakota, 8
North Lehigh Coal and Iron Police Association, 57, 58,63, 64, 65, 108; authority of, 58; massacre by, 63, 64, 65, transformation of, 108–127; weapons of, 58, 64, 65. *See also* Police, Coal and Iron
North West Detective Agency. *See* Pinkertons
Nuremburg, 117

occupation, coalfield, 52, 127–147, 185–190
Oberrender, E.A., 65, 108–126; snitches of, 108–119
Ohio, 8, 63
Ojibwe, 45
Old Forge, 116, 146
Olyphant, 146
Oneida, 116–118, 125
operators, coal: cartel of, 54–57, 140, 161; claims of poverty by, 140; concessions by, 85, 86, 89, 98, 161; demands for protection by, 12, 64, 104, 113, 131, 141, 181; depiction of miners by, 12, 27, 32, 33, 70, 102, 141, 142, 149, 172, 173, 183; employment practices of, 11, 25, 27, 28; hiring by, 11, 25 26, 28, 171; negotiation tactics of, 39, 68, 70, 81, 146–150, 161; strikebreaking strategies of, 13, 25, 36, 70, 82, 101–103, 109–127, 189, 190; use of police by, 11, 101–104 107–127, 174–178
Ottawa, 45

Paliewicz, Joseph, 133, 134
Pardee and Company, 58, 64, 152
Pardee, Frank, 163
Parker, E.W., 161, 169
patch, mine, 24, 27, 40, 58, 75, 129, 138, 153–159, 178, 190; life in a, 154-159. *See also* houses, company
Patterson, J.M, Dr., 4
peasants: Slovakian, 75; Polish, 75
Penn, Thomas, 43
Penn, William, 43
Pennsylvania, 16; claims of lawlessness in, 188; disputed origins of, 43; geography of, 22, 44; geology of, 44; settlement of, 43–46, 135, 136
Pennsylvania Federation of Labor, 184
Pennsylvania National Guard, ix; 11, 106; encampments of, 131; failures in strikes by, 12, 143–147; origins of, 181-184; strike headquarters of, 135; sympathy for strikers by, 143–145; use in strikes of, 11, 12, 106, 131, 154
Pennsylvania Railroad, 181, 191
Pennsylvania and Reading Railroad, 39
Pennypacker, Samuel, 184
Philadelphia, 48, 53–55, 58, 97–100, 101, 108, 109, 112, 131, 143, 144, 170, 185
Philadelphia and Reading Coal and Iron Company, 55, 56, 101, 131
Philadelphia and Reading Railroad, 48, 54–56; secret land purchases of, 54–56; tactics of, 54–56
Philadelphia Railroad, 182
Pinkerton, Allen, 58, 59; role in destroying unions by, 59; view of unions by, 59

Pinkerton Detective Agency, 32, 56–60, 97, 108, 113, 124, 183; investigation of Molly Maguires by, 59–61. *See also* agencies, detective
Pittsburgh, 6, 26, 80, 97
Pittsburgh Coal Company: Imperial barracks, 3; Montour Mine #9, 2; size of coalfield holdings by, 6; wages paid miners by, 6
Pittsburgh Post-Gazette, 6
Platt, Ario Pardee, 64, 110, 175–177
Plymouth, 146
Polanders, 26. *See also* miners, anthracite: slurs used against
police: blurring of line between public and private, 192; campaign to reform, 9–11; eatery, 7; efforts to abolish, 1–11, 53, 54; electric, 7; expanding discretion of, 114, 115; jurisdiction of, 114, 127, 185, 187; merchant, 7, 8; myth of accountability of, 10, 192; order mandate of, 13, 183, 185; origins of, 8–13, 57, 99, 100, 108–114, 181–193; professionalization of, 10–13, 183–193; quarry, 7; railroad, 7, 8; roadhouse, 7; role of, 10–13, 101–127, 181–193; steamboat, 7, 8; suborning perjury by, 134, 143; tactics of, 8–10, 28, 32, 56, 59, 145, 154
Police, Coal and Iron, 7–14, 36, 56, 62, 96, 97; 101, 114, 141, 149, 180, 187–92; assassination by the, 142; campaign to abolish, 9–11, 192; failures of, 12, 106, 107; powers of, 7, 53, 108, 109; recruitment of, 101; reform of, 10; statute allowing for, 7, 53, 57, 109; use of violence by, 7, 107
police, constabulary, 7, 8, 12, 26, 130, 133, 188; payment of, 8; Royal Irish, 185
police, sheriff's deputies, 1, 8, 27, 58, 114; eviction by, 154–159 192; private armies of, 11, 58, 181; strikebreaking duty by, 8, 9, 58, 63, 64; violence of, 9, 58, 63, 64. *See also* posses
police, state, 174, 178, 180; nicknames for, 186; origins of, 181–193; violence of, 185–193
Popucum, Joe, 152, 158; eviction of, 158
posses, 58, 63, 64, 65, 100; at Lattimer, 110, 175, 176, 181, 183, 187. *See also* police, sheriff's deputies
Post-Gazette, Pittsburg, 6
Pottsville, 54, 60, 120, 126, 143
Pottawatomie, 45
Powell, Thomas, 173
Price, John, 18
progressives: support of police

by, 10, 66, 67, 192
Progressive Era: origins of police in, ix, 66; role of strikes in, ix
Puerto Rico, 185
Public Safety, Committees of, 182

railroads, coal-carrying, 28, 38, 39, 55–57, 182; police and, 181, 182; preparations for strikes by, 98; strike of 1877 against, 8; transportation of coal by, 22
rafts, 22. *See also* arks
Raught, William, 65
Railway Conductors, Order of, 161
Ray, Frank, 151
Reading Railroad, 182
Revolutionary War, 185
Rhode Island, 189
Richards, Frank, 170
Ridgeway, Schuyler, 110–112
Roarity, James, 60
Rohland, Charles, 117
Ronamus, William, 142, 143
Roosevelt, Theodore, 12, 146, 149, 161, 189
Rosko, Martin, 65
rivers: development of, 43, 47, 48; shipping on, 22, 48, 50

Sacco and Vanzetti, 1
saloon, 29, 30, 32, 113, 119, 123, 125, 133, 142,
scabs, 112, 28, 29, 36, 56, 64, 70, 101, 102, 117, 118, 125, 126, 138–146, 150, 179; perjury by, 118, 125, 126; snitches and, 116–121; treatment of, 70, 103–107; use in strikes of, 64, 108–121
Schuylkill County, 40, 49–52, 56, 110, 186
Schuylkill River, 43, 46, 47
Scranton, 39, 71, 81, 131, 146, 161, 163, 181; City Guard, 182
Second City Troop of Philadelphia, 144
Seneca, 45
Shabolick, Andrew, 65
Shamokin, 38, 70, 77, 79–82, 145, 146, 179
Shafer, Ross, 3, 5
Sharpe, Patrick: assassination by police of, 141–144; martyrdom of, 143
Shawnee, 45
Shenandoah, 26, 27, 99, 106; occupation of, 129–147
Shenandoah City colliery, 132
Sheppton, 116–118, 124–126
Shovlin, Duff, 115, 116
Shovlin, Henry, 40, 151, 157; eviction of, 157
Shrader, John, 115
Silver Brook colliery, 64
Siney, John, 51, 52, 54–56, 63, 89, 94
Slapikas, Frank, 1, 2, 3, 4, 5; murder of Borcoski by, 2–6
slave patrol, 8
Slav, 26–29, 75, 130. *See also* miners, anthracite: slurs

used against
Smith, L.C., 108–112, 115, 117, 120, 124, 163
Snyder, Baird, 141
souls of capital, rotten 32, 33. *See also* bosses
South Carolina, 8
South Dakota, 8
Spalding, John L., 162, 170
Spanish American War, 110, 185
Squadron, Flying the, 100–127, 174–179, 186; arming of, 111; origins of, 108–112, role of secret service department in, 113–124, strategies of, 115, 116
Stanton colliery, 107
St. Clair, Arthur, 45
St. Clair's Defeat, 45, 46. *See also* Battle of a Thousand Slain; Battle of the Wabash River
steamships, 25
St. John, John, 184
strikebreaking, 52, 55
strikes, coal: arbitration to end, 149, 150–153, 161–180; coverage of, 11, 12, 66, 79, 80, 129, 130; fear of, 37, 82–100; funds for, 90, 145; of 1849, 50; of 1869, 52; of 1875, 56, 137, 181; of 1877, 136; of 1887, 63; of 1897, 63, 64, 185; of 1900, 36, 67, 68, 95, 96, 141, 150; of 1922, 189, 190; of 1934 by, 9; organizing for, 67, 68, 71–100; parades during, 104–106, 115, 118, 119; picketing during, 112; role in origins of police of, 12–14, 181–193; sympathy, 38; violence of police in, 12, 56, 63–64; use of strikebreakers in, 56; wildcat, 28, 55, 68, 70, 103, 179
Sugar Notch, 107
Sunbury, 135
Susquehanna River,43, 46

Tamaqua, 143, 146
temperance, 66
ton, miners', the, 21, 22, 29, 38, 164, 178; measure of, 21, 29
Tower, Charlemagne, 52

Underground Railroad, 59
United Anthracite Miners of Pennsylvania, 192
United Mine Workers of America: anti-immigrant sentiment of, 27, 67; compromise by 11, 37, 38, 51; conservative leaders of, 11, 37, 38, 51, 66, 88, 102, 190, 191; decision making methods of the, 81–100, 102, 179; demands of, 38, 51, 52, 70, 87, 150, 151, 152, 163, 164, 178; infiltration of, 37, 77, 124, 189–191; injunction against, 117; origins of, 50, 51, 63, 97; purging of radical by, 191–193; role of women in, 28, 58; strikes of, 11–13, 63, 64, 90, 145, 67–120; tactics of, 11, 51,

64, 103, 104, 139, 145; use of badges by, 79, 139

Van Wickle Coal Company, 154
Vercheck, George, 65
Vigilance and Safety, Committee of, 181
Virginia, 8, 50

Wabash River, 45
Walking Purchase, 43, 44
Wanamie, 107
War of 1812, 50, 185
Warrior Run, 107
washeries, 61, 62, 163
Washington, DC, 178
Washington, George, 45
Washington (State), 8
Waskevicz, John, 115, 116
Wassmer, Albin, 115, 118–120
watchmen, night, 8
Watkins, M.C. *See* Lyster, Walter
Watkins, Thomas H., 161
Watts, Harold, 1, 2, 3, 4, 5; murder of Borcoski by, 2–5; murder of M.C. Watkins by, 6; pistol whipping by, 3; prosecution for murder of Borcoski by, 6
Waweyapiersenwaw, 45
Waynesburg, 1
Weatherly, 116, 177
West Hazleton, 64
West Mine, 49
West Shenandoah colliery, 132
West Virginia, 8, 189
white damp, 34
Wilkes-Barre, 38, 116, 146, 150, 182, 187
Williams, Sydney, 151
Wilson, John M., 161
Wistar, Isaac J., 181
Wolverton, Simon, 108, 109, 179
Woodhicks, 46, 47
Workingmen's Benevolent Association, 51, 52, 56, 63, 84
Wright, Carroll, 140, 153
Wyndot, 45
Wyoming Valley, 52, 187

Yatesville, 187
Yavock, Paul, 65
Young, Willard, 110, 174, 177

ABOUT THE AUTHOR

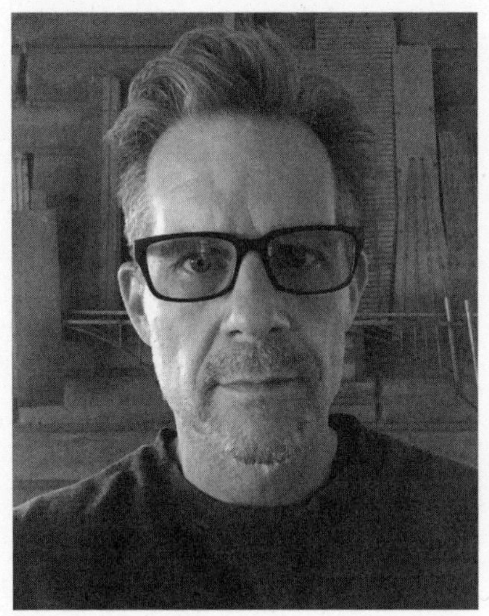

DAVID CORREIA is a professor of American Studies at the University of New Mexico. He is the author of *Properties of Violence*, coauthor with Tyler Wall of *Police: A Field Guide*, and coauthor with Nick Estes, Melanie Yazzie, and Jennifer Denetdale of *Red Nation Rising: From Bordertown Violence to Native Liberation*. With Tyler Wall he coedited *Violent Order: Essays on the Nature of Police*. He is a charter member of United Academics of the University of New Mexico, UA-UNM Local #6662.

ABOUT HAYMARKET BOOKS

Haymarket Books is a radical, independent, nonprofit book publisher based in Chicago. Our mission is to publish books that contribute to struggles for social and economic justice. We strive to make our books a vibrant and organic part of social movements and the education and development of a critical, engaged, and internationalist Left.

We take inspiration and courage from our namesakes, the Haymarket Martyrs, who gave their lives fighting for a better world. Their 1886 struggle for the eight-hour day—which gave us May Day, the international workers' holiday—reminds workers around the world that ordinary people can organize and struggle for their own liberation. These struggles—against oppression, exploitation, environmental devastation, and war—continue today across the globe.

Since our founding in 2001, Haymarket has published more than nine hundred titles. Radically independent, we seek to drive a wedge into the risk-averse world of corporate book publishing. Our authors include Angela Y. Davis, Arundhati Roy, Keeanga-Yamahtta Taylor, Eve Ewing, Aja Monet, Mariame Kaba, Naomi Klein, Rebecca Solnit, Olúfẹ́mi O. Táíwò, Mohammed El-Kurd, José Olivarez, Noam Chomsky, Winona LaDuke, Robyn Maynard, Leanne Betasamosake Simpson, Howard Zinn, Mike Davis, Marc Lamont Hill, Dave Zirin, Astra Taylor, and Amy Goodman, among many other leading writers of our time. We are also the trade publishers of the acclaimed Historical Materialism Book Series.

Haymarket also manages a vibrant community organizing and event space in Chicago, Haymarket House, the popular Haymarket Books Live event series and podcast, and the annual Socialism Conference.